SCIATICA

RELIEF WORKOUTS

For Beginners And Seniors

Effective Exercises To Alleviate Chronic Pain And Regain Independence

---

DR. THOMPSON CLARK

Disclaimer

The design of this book is centered on your health and well-being. The exercises, advice, and suggestions are intended to help you on your path to better mobility and relief. Please keep in mind, though, that every person has a unique body, so what suits one may not suit another.

Before beginning any new fitness regimen, I advise speaking with your doctor, particularly if you have any underlying medical issues or concerns. Take it slow and pay attention to your body as you go since your safety comes first.

This book is not a replacement for expert medical advice, diagnosis, or treatment; rather, it is meant to empower and inspire you with sciatica management strategies. Please contact a licensed healthcare provider if you have any questions or concerns about your health.

I hope this book gives you the inspiration, drive, and doable actions you need to live a more pleasant and active life.

Here are brief testimonies from readers who found relief and restored mobility with **"Sciatica Relief Workouts for Beginners and Seniors"**

Linda P., Denver

After years of dealing with continuous sciatica pain, I'd almost given up on finding a non-surgical treatment. I stumbled discovered this book, and it has changed my life. The exercises were straightforward, and I was able to complete them at my leisure. Within weeks, I observed a considerable drop in discomfort levels. I can now participate in things that I believed were no longer possible. Thank you.

Samuel T., Leeds

I was hesitant at first because I'd tried many different workouts and therapies for my sciatica, but this book genuinely helped. The layout of the activities made them simple to follow, especially for those with little expertise. The individualized workouts helped me restore strength and flexibility, and I can now move without concern of being in pain. This book has truly restored my confidence.

Cheryl R. and Austin

I had been suffering from sciatica on and off for years, and it only got worse as I got older. After trying the exercises in this book, I observed a slow but significant improvement. The author's observations and gentle advice made it easy for me to establish a regular regimen. I can now walk longer distances and sleep better without having to continually shift around to reach a comfortable posture.

Oliver W., Birmingham

This book was recommended to me by a friend who had found relief for her sciatica. I didn't have high expectations at first, but the exercises are simple and effective, especially for someone like me who has no fitness history. I can't believe how much of a difference it has made—not only in pain management but also in making me feel stronger and more in control of my body. Highly recommended!

Each of these readers achieved long-term relief from the book's systematic method, and their tales demonstrate how effective this program can be for anyone suffering from sciatica.

TABLE OF CONTENTS

ABOUT THE AUTHOR

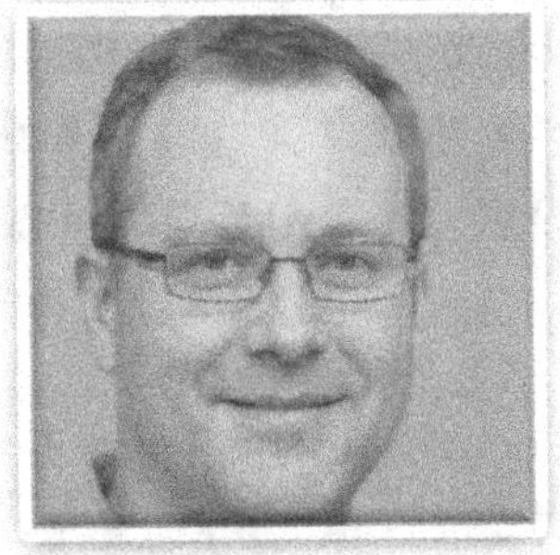

Dr. Thompson Clark is a seasoned physical therapist and geriatric care specialist with over 30 years of experience working to improve the lives of older individuals. Dr. Clark, a specialist in mobility, flexibility, and pain treatment, has established himself as a respected figure in senior health, advocating for non-invasive approaches that assist older people in preserving their freedom. His desire to help seniors stay active and healthy has led him to create simple stretching routines adapted to their specific needs.

Dr. Clark's schooling includes a *Doctorate of Physical Therapy (DPT)* with a focus on geriatric care. Early in his work, he noticed a void in elder healthcare: exercise and mobility were frequently disregarded in favor of medication or surgery. In response, he developed individualized programs to manage chronic pain, flexibility, and posture, allowing individuals of all ages to enjoy pain-free, satisfying lives. His method emphasizes the importance of simple, effective exercises that anyone can undertake, regardless of fitness level.

As an author, Dr. Clark has written extensively about senior health and wellness, making complicated medical concepts simple for his readers. His books and articles highlight the benefits of stretching and movement for older people, providing practical recommendations that seniors can adopt into their everyday routines. His writing has a devoted audience due to his ability to explain health information without compromising depth or accuracy.

In addition to his professional practice and writing, Dr. Clark is a prominent advocate for seniors' mental and emotional well-being. He incorporates mindfulness and relaxation techniques into his stretching sessions, which assist older folks manage stress and anxiety while improving their physical health. His holistic approach emphasizes the link between mind and body, encouraging elders to look after both parts of their well-being.

Dr. Clark is active in his community, providing free workshops and wellness initiatives for seniors, particularly in impoverished regions. His dedication to keeping older individuals active and healthy extends beyond his professional career, as he continues to educate healthcare workers and promote wellness programs that enable seniors to live their best lives.

INTRODUCTION

I recall when I first met Clara Montgomery. She was not one of my regular patients, but rather an unexpected visitor to the local coffee shop in Wichita, Kansas. She went in with a little limp, her gaze surveying the room as if the entire world rested on her shoulders. I noted the pain on her face, which felt both familiar to me as a health practitioner and uniquely personal to her.

Clara was just in her mid-50s, but it was evident she was suffering from sciatica. She sat down, ordered a cappuccino, and winced slightly, correcting her position before sighing softly. I could see the discomfort that every slightest movement seemed to cause. It was a sense I'd felt before, but something about Clara's energy made me believe this story would be unique.

Over the next three days, I ran into Clara again. This time, I chose to introduce myself. I smiled warmly and suggested that join her for coffee. She agreed, and we started talking right away. Clara didn't take long to give me her story.

"I've had sciatica for years," she remarked quietly, her fingers circling the lip of her coffee cup. *"It began in my early 40s, but it gradually worsened. Some days, I can't walk without feeling like my leg is going to give out. The doctor indicated I needed surgery, but I'm not sure I can go through with it. So, for the*

Her words struck home. I'd heard similar stories before, stories of chronic pain that hampered so many people's lives, particularly those who had been suffering from sciatica for years. Clara attempted a variety of remedies, but nothing seemed to stick. Pills provided momentary relief, but nothing addressed the underlying source of her suffering. Surgery loomed in the distance like a dark cloud, an option she wasn't yet ready to confront.

"I've tried several things," she explained, "but nothing has truly worked for me. I know I should move and stretch, but it might feel overwhelming at times. "I don't know where to begin."

Over the sound of coffee cups clinking and the low hum of the cafe, I realized Clara was looking for more than just advice. She needed to get out of the cycle of misery and frustration. She required a guide, someone who could show her how to overcome the anguish and restore her independence.

That's when I told her about the book ***"Sciatica Relief Workouts for Beginners and Seniors"*** I'd been working on. I had been working on a program of mild, effective exercises that I had observed benefit many people, including Clara. These movements were not intended to push through discomfort, but rather to restore the body's natural equilibrium and relieve strain on the sciatic nerve. They concentrated on *FLEXIBILITY, STRENGTH, AND POSTURE,* three important factors that could alleviate her pain and help her regain control of her body.

Clara was fascinated, but skeptical. She had tried innumerable things previously, and it appeared almost too simple to be true. But I informed her, and I will guarantee you now, that the trip she was about to embark on was not about radical, overnight changes, but rather incremental, achievable measures that would lead to long-term outcomes. I told her how many people, like her, had found relief and healing from similar exercises.

*Take **Tommy** for example. Tommy, a dedicated truck driver from the nearby town of El Dorado, has been suffering from sciatica for nearly ten years. He was in his mid-60s and had tried everything, including cortisone shots, physical therapy, and a brief effort at acupuncture. Nothing brought him lasting relief. Tommy noticed a difference after only a few weeks of incorporating some of the program's workouts. He was able to get out of bed without grimacing in agony, and he began walking again without the use of a cane. It was not a miracle; it was a combination of constancy, patience, and a small amount of dedication to change.*

I told Clara Tommy's story, and I saw hope in her eyes. It wasn't the hope of a speedy repair, but rather the hope that comes from knowing there is a way forward. She did not have to live in pain indefinitely, and she did not require surgery to regain control of her health.

Clara began her adventure. Every day, she included stretches, light strength exercises, and balance routines in her workout. Initially, it was challenging. She became frustrated on occasion, but she persevered. She gradually noticed little changes, such as less pain while sitting and less stiffness when standing. The exercises, which she had felt were too simple to make a difference, were her lifeline.

Clara quickly noticed the improvements in other areas of her life. She regained her confidence, began walking greater distances, and found herself moving more comfortably. The changes were not dramatic, but they were real, and they reinforced one another. What began as a simple step towards relief evolved into a new way of life.

This book is the guide I wish I had given Clara from the start. It's a compilation of tried-and-true exercises and tactics that can help you break free from the cycle of chronic pain and regain control of your life. These exercises are for you, whether you've had sciatica for years or are just starting to notice symptoms. They are easy, effective, and, most importantly, are intended to benefit your long-term health.

You, like Clara, can restore your independence, minimize your pain, and feel more secure in your body. The trip may not always be simple, but with perseverance, patience, and the appropriate approach, you will begin to see results. This book will help you get out of bed without grimacing, walk without discomfort, and enjoy life without chronic pain.

So, I invite you to take the initial step, as Clara did. It will not be the easiest journey you've ever taken, but it will be one of the most fulfilling. Let us embark on this path together, you deserve to live without the continual shadow of misery hanging over you.

CHAPTER 1: UNDERSTANDING SCIATICA AND THE CAUSES

What Is Sciatica? A Summary Of Symptoms And Pain Patterns

Sciatica is a phrase used to describe pain that spreads down the length of the sciatic nerve, the body's longest and broadest nerve. This nerve originates in the lower spine, travels down the hips and buttocks, and then down each leg, branching into smaller nerves that reach the toes. Sciatica pain is normally limited to one side of the body and is caused by compression, irritation, or inflammation of the sciatic nerve. Understanding sciatica necessitates knowledge of its symptoms, pain patterns, underlying causes, and how the body reacts to this type of nerve pain.

What Causes Sciatica?

Sciatica is a sign of anything compressing or aggravating the sciatic nerve, not an illness in and of itself. Sciatica can be caused by a variety of factors, most commonly structural or degenerative abnormalities in the spine or surrounding tissues. Each reason produces a unique set of pain patterns and consequences, depending on the location and intensity of the nerve compression. *Here's a more detailed look at the basic causes of sciatica.*

1. Herniated or Slipped Disc

Sciatica is commonly caused by a herniated disc, also known as a slipped or burst disc. Discs in the spine function as cushions between vertebrae, allowing for smooth movement and absorbing shock. These discs feature a soft, gel-like core (nucleus) and a harder outer layer (annulus).

Disc herniation occurs when the annulus tears or weakens, allowing the soft nucleus to bulge or ooze out and impinge on adjacent nerves. A herniated disc in the lower back (lumbar spine), where the sciatic nerve roots are located, can compress the nerve directly, causing pain to radiate down the leg.

Disc herniation is frequently caused by gradual wear and tear, or disc degeneration. As we get older, the discs lose water content, become less flexible, and are more prone to tearing when under pressure or strain. In younger people, herniation can occur as a result of acute injuries from carrying large objects incorrectly, sports injuries, or even awkward motions.

2. Spinal Stenosis

Spinal stenosis is a narrowing of the gaps within the spine that can cause pressure on the spinal cord and nerve roots, especially the sciatic nerve. It primarily affects older persons, as aging can cause spinal structures to morph and shift.

Lumbar spinal stenosis, which causes narrowing in the lower back, is the most frequent cause of sciatica. Cervical spinal stenosis, which affects the neck, does not usually induce sciatica symptoms. As people age, arthritis, thicker ligaments, and bone spurs (abnormal bony growths) can cause spinal stenosis.

These modifications may restrict the spinal canal or foramina (openings where nerves escape), squeezing the sciatic nerve roots. Spinal stenosis symptoms include numbness, tingling, and weakness, which can increase over time. In severe cases, it might cause balance and movement difficulties.

3. Piriformis Syndrome

Piriformis syndrome develops when the piriformis muscle, a tiny muscle deep in the buttocks, spasms or contracts, pressing on the sciatic nerve. The sciatic nerve is quite close to the piriformis muscle, and in rare cases, it even crosses through it. If the piriformis becomes inflamed or tight, it can irritate or compress the sciatic nerve, resulting in sciatica-like discomfort.

Piriformis syndrome can be caused by extended sitting, repetitive lower-body exercises (such as jogging or cycling), or injuries from falls. Poor posture and inappropriate stretching or warm-up regimens can potentially strain the piriformis muscle.

Unlike classic sciatica, which begins in the lumbar back, piriformis syndrome commonly causes buttock discomfort that can go down the leg. It is sometimes known as "pseudo-sciatica" since it involves muscular discomfort rather than direct nerve compression.

4. Degenerative Disc Disease

Degenerative disc disease is a condition in which the spinal discs gradually degrade, losing their cushioning function and causing spinal instability. Although this is a typical component of the aging process, excessive degradation might result in symptoms.

As a disc loses height and shape, the space between vertebrae narrows. This loss of height can increase pressure on surrounding nerves, especially the sciatic nerve, causing sciatica symptoms. As the body attempts to stabilize the spine, bone spurs may form around the degenerative disc. These spurs might restrict the spinal canal and crush nerve roots.

Common risk factors for degenerative disc disease include age, heredity, past injuries, and repetitive strain. The issue is more common in people over the age of 50 and can lead to chronic lower back pain and sciatica.

5. Injury or Trauma

Physical injuries to the lower back, hips, or legs can result in sciatica by creating structural abnormalities or inflammation that irritate the nerve. Sudden impacts from falls, automobile accidents, or sports injuries can dislocate vertebrae or induce soft tissue edema, compressing the sciatic nerve.

Lifting heavy objects incorrectly or repeatedly over time can strain the lower back, resulting in herniated discs or other spinal misalignments that can impact the sciatic nerve. Severe muscle strains or spasms in the lower back or buttocks can cause the sciatic nerve to be compressed or irritated. While less prevalent, soft tissue injuries can occasionally cause sciatic pain.

6. Bone Spurs and Osteoarthritis

Osteoarthritis, a degenerative joint disease, can cause bone spurs, which are bony growths that occur along the borders of bones. These growths can put pressure on the sciatic nerve, producing pain and discomfort. As osteoarthritis causes cartilage in joints to deteriorate, bones may rub together. The body compensates by growing bone spurs, which can restrict space in the spinal canal and foramina, squeezing nerves.

Bone spurs in the lumbar spine can directly compress the sciatic nerve roots, causing discomfort to spread down the leg. Symptoms may also include stiffness, numbness, and restricted mobility. Aging, obesity, genetic susceptibility, and previous accidents all raise the risk of developing osteoarthritis and bone spurs, which can lead to sciatica.

7. Spondylolisthesis

Spondylolisthesis occurs when one vertebra moves forward over the vertebra below it. This slippage can compress the sciatic nerve, resulting in sciatica. This disorder can be congenital (existing at birth) or develop later as a result of age-related degeneration, trauma, or repetitive strain. It is more common in the lower spine (lumbar area), which increases the likelihood of sciatic nerve compression.

Symptoms of spondylolisthesis include lower back discomfort, leg pain, muscular stiffness, and leg weakness. Sciatica symptoms usually worsen after prolonged physical activity, such as walking or standing.

People with a history of spinal injuries, athletes who engage in repetitive spinal strain (e.g., gymnasts, weightlifters), and older adults with degenerative changes in the spine are also at higher risk.

8. Tumors or Infections

Although rare, spinal tumors and infections can cause sciatica by putting pressure on the sciatic nerve or its root. Spinal tumors can compress the sciatic nerve, causing pain and other neurological symptoms. The risk is quite low, but a tumor should be explored if sciatica arises unexpectedly without a clear mechanical explanation.

Infections in the spine or surrounding tissues can produce inflammation and edema, potentially irritating the sciatic nerve. Spinal abscesses and osteomyelitis (bone infection) are rare, but they can cause sciatic pain.

When sciatica is caused by tumors or infections, the pain may be accompanied by additional symptoms including fever, unexplained weight loss, or night sweats. Prompt medical intervention is required to rule out these dangerous conditions.

9. Pregnancy

Pregnancy can cause transient sciatica because of increased weight, altered posture, and changes in the center of gravity. As the baby grows, the extra weight and strain on the lower back and pelvis can compress the sciatic nerve. Furthermore, hormonal changes during pregnancy lead joints and ligaments to loosen, which can put extra strain on the spine.

Pregnant women with sciatica may suffer pain spreading from the lower back to their buttocks and legs. The pain is usually just transient and subsides after delivery. Gentle exercise, stretching, and posture adjustments can help alleviate sciatic pain during pregnancy.

Symptoms Of Sciatica

Sciatica causes a wide range of symptoms, from slight discomfort to severe, crippling pain. The symptoms of sciatica differ from those of other types of lower back pain in that they follow the path of the sciatic nerve, which extends from the lower back to the hips and buttocks and down each leg. These symptoms can affect one or both legs, and the severity varies depending on the underlying reason for the nerve compression.

Let's look at some of the most prevalent sciatica symptoms:

1. Radiating pain along the sciatic nerve pathway

Radiating pain is the primary sign of sciatica. Sciatica pain usually starts in the lower back and moves down one leg along the sciatic nerve. It can impact the nerve's whole route, which includes the hip, buttocks, thigh, knee, calf, ankle, and even the foot. The majority of persons with sciatica begin to feel discomfort in the lower back, where the sciatic nerve originates. This pain may present as a mild aching or tightness, but it can develop over time.

Sciatica can cause pain in the buttocks, which is one of the first locations to be impacted. Buttock pain may indicate that the sciatic nerve is inflamed or compressed in the lumbar spine or pelvis. The pain may feel like soreness or heaviness that worsens after sitting or standing for an extended amount of time.

As the nerve travels down the leg, pain often follows. The pain often follows the path of the sciatic nerve, which runs from the lower back to the buttocks and down the back of the thigh, knee, calf, and foot. In severe situations, the pain can extend to the toes. This radiating pain might be severe, scorching, or stabbing in character, and it can even seem like an electrical shock.

2. Sharp, burning, or shooting pain

Sciatica is commonly described as a sharp, shooting pain that travels from the lower back down the leg. The pain can feel like a burning feeling or a strong discomfort, comparable to that caused by a pinched nerve. This sort of pain can occur quickly and intensely, making it difficult to move or even find a comfortable position.

Shooting pain is a rapid, acute, and sharp pain that goes fast down the leg, usually produced by movements like standing up, leaning forward, or raising. The sensation of burning in the leg can be akin to a muscle cramp or severe muscle tension and create significant discomfort.

3. Numbness and tingling

In addition to pain, many people with sciatica have numbness or tingling along the route of the sciatic nerve. This sensation, often known as pins and needles, might be especially evident in the lower leg, ankle, or foot. Numbness and tingling occur when the sciatic nerve is compressed or inflamed, interfering with the normal passage of nervous impulses.

Pins and needles are the sensation of tiny, sharp pricks or tingling caused by nerve compression or inflammation in the affected leg. Numbness is a loss of sensation or a sense of "deadness" in the leg or foot that can make it difficult to feel objects or move the affected body parts normally.

4. Muscle Weakness

Sciatica may also induce muscle weakness in the afflicted leg. This occurs when nerve compression impairs the sciatic nerve's capacity to signal muscles to contract properly. Individuals may notice that their leg feels weak or that they have difficulty lifting their feet or bending their knees. Muscle weakness can make it difficult to stand, walk, and climb stairs.

One of the earliest indicators of muscle weakening is the inability to lift the leg, particularly the foot, off the floor. This is also known as foot drop, which occurs when the foot drags or catches on the ground due to weakness in the muscles controlled by the sciatic nerve. As muscle weakness develops, actions such as walking, sitting, standing, and lifting become increasingly difficult. This can have a substantial impact on movement and balance.

5. Pain that worsens after certain movements

Sciatica pain frequently worsens with specific activities or motions that put greater strain on the sciatic nerve or lower back. *Common actions that can worsen sciatica pain include:*

❖ Bending or twisting: Any forward or backward bending or twisting motions can put pressure on the spine, aggravating the nerve and exacerbating the discomfort.

❖ Prolonged sitting: Sitting for lengthy periods, particularly on hard surfaces, can place stress on the sciatic nerve. This is especially common among those who work from a desk or drive for long periods. Sitting in poor posture or slumping forward can exacerbate the discomfort.

❖ Lifting or carrying heavy objects: Lifting or straining the lower back in any way can compress the spine and worsen sciatic pain, resulting in acute or shooting pains.

❖ Coughing or sneezing can put unexpected pressure on the lower spine, exacerbating sciatica symptoms for a short time.

6. Pain Relief from certain positions

Some sciatica sufferers discover that particular positions or motions alleviate their discomfort. These positions typically minimize pressure on the sciatic nerve and relieve compression. *For example:*

❖ Lying down with knees bent can help reduce pressure on the lower spine. This position is usually recommended for people who have sciatica discomfort.

❖ Elevating the legs: While sitting or lying down, elevate your legs up on a stool or pillow to relieve strain on the sciatic nerve.

7. Loss of reflexes

In more severe episodes of sciatica, compression of the sciatic nerve can cause reflex loss in the affected limb. This occurs because the sciatic nerve regulates certain reflexes in the knee and ankle. Loss of reflexes can be detected during a physical examination and indicate that nerve compression has progressed to a more significant degree.

The knee jerk reflex may be reduced or absent due to nerve compression in the lower spine.

Ankle reflex: The ankle jerk reflex may also be impaired, causing difficulty standing on tiptoe or elevating the foot.

8. Bilateral sciatica (rare)

Sciatica can sometimes affect both legs at once. This ailment, known as bilateral sciatica, usually indicates a more serious underlying issue, such as spinal stenosis, a ruptured disc, or a tumor pressing on the spinal cord. Bilateral sciatica may cause more severe mobility problems and necessitate rapid medical intervention.

When sciatica strikes both legs, the pain may be less localized and more broad, making it difficult to pinpoint the exact site of discomfort.

9. Cauda equina syndrome (Emergency)

Sciatica can be an indication of cauda equina syndrome, a serious disorder caused by significant nerve compression at the base of the spinal cord. This illness necessitates rapid medical attention and might result in irreversible damage if not handled promptly.

Symptoms of cauda equina syndrome include bladder or bowel control problems, sexual dysfunction, and abrupt paralysis in both legs. Cauda equina syndrome can also cause severe, persistent lower back discomfort and groin numbness (known as saddle anesthesia).

Sciatica symptoms vary from person to person, but the most typical feature is pain radiating from the lower back down one leg, usually along the sciatic nerve. The level of this discomfort varies, from subtle aches to acute, shooting pains. Other symptoms could include numbness, tingling, muscle weakness, and pain that intensifies with certain motions or positions. Understanding these symptoms is crucial for seeking appropriate therapy and effectively managing sciatica. If the symptoms worsen or do not improve with conservative care, it is critical to seek medical attention to ensure adequate treatment and avoid long-term problems.

Pain Patterns In Sciatica

Sciatica pain can vary in kind and location based on the underlying cause of the ailment, the level of nerve involvement, and personal characteristics such as posture and physical activity. The pain patterns in sciatica are critical for evaluating the condition's evolution and choosing the best treatments.

Here's a closer look at the various pain patterns connected with sciatica:

1. Pain begins in the lower back and buttocks

The pain usually starts in the lower back or buttocks and radiates down the leg. In the early stages of sciatica, people may experience a dull, agonizing pain in their lower back. The first pain may be aggravated with specific activities, such as bending, lifting, or twisting. As the pressure on the sciatic nerve grows, the pain may shift and radiate downward along its route.

Throbbing or dull ache is prevalent in the early stages of sciatica and may appear as a continual background discomfort. Increased intensity when performing specific actions, such as bending forward, twisting the spine, or lifting objects. Pain may migrate to the buttocks or hips, impacting the hip flexors and glutes.

This type of pain is frequently caused by disorders such as degenerative disc degeneration, lumbar spinal stenosis, or sacroiliac joint dysfunction, in which the compression or irritation begins at the lower lumbar spine (L3 to L5) and spreads downward.

2. Radiating pain down the back of the leg

As sciatica worsens, pain often travels down the back of the leg. This is one of the classic symptoms of sciatica, and it frequently worsens with movement or prolonged positions that put pressure on the sciatic nerve. The discomfort may begin in the lower back or buttocks and progress down the thigh, calf, and even to the foot or toe.

The pain may be similar to an electric shock or a deep, stabbing sensation traveling down the back of the leg. As the nerve travels through the gluteal muscles and thigh, discomfort typically radiates to the back of the leg, making it difficult to stand or walk comfortably. In extreme cases, pain can radiate down the calf, ankle, and foot, typically worsening with movement, walking, or extended standing.

Pain radiating down the leg is often associated with herniated discs or lumbar stenosis, in which a herniated or degenerating disc pushes on the sciatic nerve. The severity of the pain varies according to the degree of compression.

3. Pain radiating to the calves and feet

Some people with sciatica experience pain radiating down to the calf, ankle, and sometimes the toes. This form of discomfort is usually more severe and can significantly impede mobility. In addition to the acute, shooting pain, people may feel numbness, tingling, or a "pins and needles" sensation that spreads to their feet. This pattern develops when nerve compression affects the lower parts of the sciatic nerve, such as the S1 nerve root, which controls the muscles of the foot and lower leg.

Flexing or extending the foot, such as while walking or standing on tiptoes, might aggravate the pain or cause intense discomfort in the calf or foot. In severe situations, the pain may make it difficult to walk, stand, or lift the foot, greatly impairing daily activities.

This pain pattern is frequently associated with illnesses such as sciatica produced by a herniated disc, in which the disc compresses the nerve roots that supply sensation and motor control to the lower leg and foot.

4. Pain worse by sitting, bending, or twisting

Long periods of sitting are one of the most prominent causes of sciatica pain. Sitting puts pressure on the sciatic nerve, particularly in the lower back and buttocks, causing discomfort to travel down the leg. Actions such as bending, twisting, or lifting can exacerbate the pain by putting additional strain on the afflicted discs, muscles, or joints.

People suffering from sciatica may discover that sitting for lengthy periods (such as during vehicle journeys or at a desk) initiates or intensifies their pain, especially if they sit with bad posture. Activities such as picking something up from the ground, twisting to reach for an object, and even some yoga postures can aggravate sciatic pain. These movements put more pressure on the spinal discs or compress the muscles and joints that press on the nerves.

Standing or walking can help relieve pain because it distributes pressure away from the nerve. However, extended walking might increase the pain if it puts a constant strain on the lower back. This pain pattern is frequently associated with disorders such as herniated discs or lumbar spinal stenosis, in which nerve root compression generates pain that intensifies with specific motions.

5. Bilateral pain (pain on both sides)

Though sciatica usually affects one side of the body, in rare situations, people may have pain on both sides, which is known as bilateral sciatica. This uncommon type of sciatica frequently indicates more serious underlying disorders, such as a massive herniated disc, spinal stenosis, or cauda equina syndrome, which involves compression of the nerve roots at the base of the spine.

Individuals with bilateral sciatica may experience pain in both their lower back and legs. This can make it difficult to walk and keep balance. Bilateral sciatica is frequently linked with more extreme pain and can be followed by other symptoms such as limb weakness or numbness, which impede daily activities. Neurological symptoms include bowel or bladder problems (incontinence or retention), which can indicate a medical emergency such as cauda equina syndrome.

6. Numbness, tingling, or "pins and needles"

In addition to discomfort, sciatica can induce numbness, tingling, or "pins and needles" throughout the nerve pathway. This is most commonly seen in the leg or foot and is caused by nerve compression or irritation. While pain is frequently the most visible sign, sensory abnormalities can also be debilitating, interfering with movement and function.

The affected leg or foot may feel "dead" or "numb," making it difficult to detect temperature or pressure changes. Numbness and tingling can impair balance and coordination, making it difficult to walk or move without falling.

This sensory disturbance is produced by pressure on the sciatic nerve, which impairs the nerve's capacity to convey sensory signals properly. It is usually associated with disorders such as lumbar disc herniation and spinal stenosis.

Sciatica pain varies in intensity, location, and duration according to the individual and the underlying cause of nerve compression. Pain can spread from the lower back to the buttocks, down the back of the leg, and even to the foot, and is frequently increased by specific motions or extended sitting. Understanding these pain patterns is critical for diagnosing the underlying disease and choosing the most effective therapies, such as physical therapy, stretching, or more advanced medical interventions. Sciatica can worsen over time if not treated, so early intervention is critical for treating the illness and increasing quality of life.

How Sciatica Impacts Daily Life

Sciatica's pain, numbness, tingling, and weakness can make even simple chores difficult, creating both physical and mental misery. The severity of sciatica symptoms varies from person to person, but for many, it is an ongoing struggle to manage and live with.

1. Pain Interrupts Routine Movements

One of the most disruptive parts of sciatica is the pain it generates, which can make even simple movements extremely difficult. The sciatic nerve goes from the lower back, down the buttocks, and through the back of the legs, hence the pain is typically felt during routine activities such as:

❖ Bending: Bending over to tie shoes, pick something up, or even tie a child's shoelaces can cause severe discomfort. Bending needs the lower back and hips to flex, which puts pressure on the sciatic nerve and worsens discomfort.

❖ Twisting: Activities such as looking over your shoulder while driving or reaching in a different direction might irritate the sciatic nerve. Twisting motions put tension on the lower spine's muscles and discs, potentially worsening nerve compression.

❖ Lifting: Picking up objects, especially heavy or strangely shaped ones, can put a strain on the spine and sciatic nerve, exacerbating the pain. Even something as simple as lifting a grocery bag might cause pain for those with sciatica.

2. Walking and Mobility Challenges

Walking is an essential part of daily life, but for persons with sciatica, it may be a painful agony. The discomfort usually extends down one side of the body, making every step more difficult. The discomfort may begin as a minor ache but can quickly escalate into a strong, shooting feeling that impairs one's ability to walk for extended periods.

Some people with sciatica develop a limp to avoid putting weight on the affected leg, which can lead to additional issues such as:

❖ Postural imbalances: Shifting weight to the opposite leg to compensate for pain can produce misalignments in the spine, hips, and pelvis, resulting in extra discomfort and muscle tension in other sections of the body.

❖ Reduced endurance: Walking longer distances or standing for extended periods of time can be exhausting owing to pain. This can have a significant impact on a person's capacity to carry out regular tasks such as grocery shopping, running errands, and even attending social events.

❖ Reduced mobility: People with severe sciatica may avoid walking altogether to avoid causing discomfort. This constraint can create a vicious cycle, resulting in decreased physical activity, muscle weakening, and even joint stiffness, exacerbating mobility concerns.

3. Sitting and Resting Difficulties

Sitting for long periods can be one of the most painful activities for people who have sciatica. Whether at a desk, in the car, or at the dining table, the strain on the spine and sciatic nerve can quickly produce discomfort. This occurs when sitting compresses the discs in the spine, perhaps increasing pressure on the nerve roots that contribute to sciatica. *The following are some of the most common seating challenges:*

❖ Finding a comfortable position: Many people with sciatica must experiment with different seated positions, cushions, or chairs to relieve pressure on the sciatic nerve. However, most positions only offer momentary relief, making it difficult to concentrate on work, socializing, or relaxing.

❖ Limited job productivity: People who sit at desks for work or school may have difficulty concentrating or maintaining productivity owing to pain or discomfort from prolonged sitting. Desk workers or students with sciatica may need to take more frequent breaks to stretch or stand, disturbing their daily routine.

❖ Difficulty driving: Sitting in a car for extended periods can be difficult, especially on long trips. Sciatica pain can worsen with prolonged sitting and may cause leg numbness or weakness, making it difficult to drive safely. Frequent stops, changing positions, and adjusting the car seat for comfort may be necessary, but these only provide partial relief.

4. Sleeping Troubles

People suffering from sciatica frequently experience poor sleep quality. The pain might hinder patients from finding a comfortable sleeping position, resulting in restless nights and daytime tiredness. Sciatica can influence sleep in several ways, including:

❖ Inability to lie down comfortably: Sciatica can make it difficult to lie flat on the back or side since these postures put additional strain on the sciatic nerve. The discomfort may escalate as a person changes positions or transfers their weight in an attempt to get comfortable.

❖ Frequent night waking: Sciatica can disrupt sleep patterns by generating pain or discomfort, resulting in frequent awakenings. This might lead to interrupted sleep, increasing daytime weariness and irritation.

❖ Sleep posture: Some people with sciatica find it more pleasant to sleep in a reclined position or with a pillow between their legs, although these adjustments are not always effective. People may need to sleep in a semi-sitting position to relieve pressure on the nerve, which can cause neck and back pain.

❖ Chronic fatigue: Inadequate sleep can cause chronic weariness, making it difficult to operate during the day. Fatigue can exacerbate other elements of daily living, resulting in decreased motivation and emotional stress.

5. Emotional and Mental Impact

Living with persistent pain, such as sciatica, can take a significant emotional and mental toll. Chronic pain can cause feelings of irritation, powerlessness, and anxiety. Sciatica's limits may cause a sense of loss of control, particularly if the person was previously physically active or independent.

❖ Increased stress: Constant agony from sciatica can raise stress levels, making it much more difficult to manage the pain. This can lead to feelings of despondency, which can harm both physical and mental health.

❖ Mental exhaustion: Constantly managing pain or suffering throughout the day can lead to mental fatigue. Sciatica patients may struggle to concentrate or focus on tasks owing to continuous pain.

❖ Social withdrawal: Sciatica can interfere with social activities, leading to isolation and loneliness. People may avoid social meetings or group exercise because they are in discomfort or embarrassed about their illness.

❖ Mood disturbances: Chronic pain has been related to an increased risk of depression and anxiety, as persistent discomfort can hurt a person's mental health. Feelings of irritation, worry, or melancholy are frequent, especially if sciatica interferes with everyday tasks or personal objectives.

6. Reduced Physical Activity and Fitness

A person suffering from sciatica may become less active owing to discomfort, which can lead to a vicious cycle of declining fitness over time. Reduced physical activity may:

❖ Lead to weight gain: When pain inhibits regular activity, weight management becomes more difficult. Weight gain can exacerbate sciatica pain by putting additional strain on the lower back and spine.

❖ Increased muscle weakness: When people neglect physical activity, the muscles that support their spine and core weaken. This diminishes the body's ability to stabilize the spine, resulting in increased pressure on the sciatic nerve and aggravating symptoms.

❖ Limit rehabilitation: While physical treatment and regular exercise are essential for sciatica relief, people in pain may skip these activities entirely. This can delay recovery and prevent complete rehabilitation.

7. Strain on Daily Tasks and Responsibilities

Sciatica can interfere with vital daily tasks such as caring for family members, cleaning the house, and going to work. Lifting groceries, carrying laundry, or even caring for children or pets might be difficult and unpleasant, forcing you to seek assistance from others. The inability to complete these daily duties can lead to emotions of frustration and dependency, lowering self-esteem and quality of life.

Sciatica can be a life-changing ailment that affects both physical and emotional health. Sciatica discomfort and limits can affect almost every part of everyday life, from simple movements like walking and sitting to more sophisticated activities such as working, socializing, and caring for others. Understanding these issues is critical for creating effective management methods, including exercising, maintaining correct posture, and getting medical attention when necessary. Sciatica patients can regain their independence and quality of life with the proper therapy and assistance.

Seeking Medical Attention For Sciatica

While mild cases of sciatica can be treated at home with rest, stretching, and over-the-counter medications, more severe or persistent cases often necessitate medical evaluation and intervention. The decision to seek medical attention is based on the severity, duration, and nature of the symptoms. In some cases, immediate medical attention is required to address underlying conditions, prevent worsening symptoms, and ensure the best possible outcome for the patient.

When should I seek medical attention for sciatica?

1. Severe, unrelenting pain

If sciatica pain persists despite basic self-care measures (such as rest, ice, heat, and pain relievers), it is time to see a doctor. Sciatica pain that lasts for several weeks or worsens over time, despite efforts to relieve it, may indicate that the underlying cause is more serious or necessitates different treatment approaches. Constant pain can have a significant impact on quality of life and may require medical intervention to alleviate discomfort and prevent further complications.

For example, if sitting, standing, or walking becomes unbearable despite your best efforts to manage the pain, or if the pain interferes with your ability to perform daily tasks, you must seek medical attention.

2. Numbness or weakness in the legs or feet

One of the most concerning sciatica symptoms is numbness or weakness in the affected leg or foot. Sciatica frequently causes tingling or a "pins and needles" sensation along the leg; however, if you experience a complete lack of sensation, or if your leg becomes weak and difficult to move, this may indicate nerve damage or compression. Weakness in the leg, particularly when it impairs your ability to stand or walk, may indicate that the sciatic nerve is compressed to the point where it could cause permanent damage if not treated.

In such cases, medical professionals may administer neurological tests to evaluate motor function and determine the extent of nerve involvement. Addressing this issue early can help to prevent further nerve damage and restore function.

3. Loss of bladder and bowel control

One of the most urgent and potentially serious symptoms that necessitate immediate medical attention is the loss of bladder or bowel control, also known as cauda equina syndrome. The cauda equina is a bundle of nerves at the spinal cord's end that regulates bladder, bowel, and sexual organ function. Compression or damage to this nerve bundle can result in loss of control over urination and defecation, as well as sexual dysfunction.

This is a medical emergency that requires immediate attention to avoid permanent disability. If you experience symptoms such as incontinence, a sudden inability to urinate or empty your bowels, or groin numbness, seek medical attention immediately. Surgical intervention may be required to relieve pressure on the nerves and prevent permanent damage.

4. Sudden, intense pain, or pain following an injury

If sciatica pain occurs suddenly after a traumatic injury, such as a fall, car accident, or sports injury, it is critical to seek medical attention right away. Acute injuries can result in herniated discs, fractures, or other spinal damage that necessitates immediate medical attention. Sudden, severe pain following an injury may indicate a serious spinal issue, and it is critical to seek an accurate diagnosis from a healthcare provider to determine the best treatment plan.

In cases of trauma, diagnostic imaging such as X-rays, MRIs, or CT scans may be required to assess the extent of the injury and determine the underlying cause of sciatica. Early detection and intervention can help avoid long-term complications.

5. Fever and unexpected weight loss

In rare cases, sciatica pain may be caused by infections or cancer, which can irritate the sciatic nerve. If you have sciatica and other symptoms like fever, chills, or unexplained weight loss, you should see a doctor right away. These additional symptoms may indicate an infection, tumor, or another serious medical condition affecting the spine or surrounding structures.

If sciatica pain is accompanied by these symptoms, seek immediate medical attention to rule out infections such as spinal abscesses or conditions like spinal tumors or cancer. Delaying medical attention may result in additional complications and more aggressive treatment down the line.

What to expect during a medical consultation for sciatica

When you seek medical treatment for sciatica, your doctor will conduct a thorough examination to determine the cause and severity of the problem. The assessment typically includes the following steps:

1. Medical history and symptom review

The healthcare provider will start by asking about your symptoms, such as the onset, location, and intensity of the pain, as well as any other associated symptoms like weakness, numbness, or changes in bowel or bladder function. It is critical to provide as much information as possible about when the pain began, what activities worsened it, and what provides relief. In addition, the provider will inquire about your medical history, including any previous back issues, injuries, or chronic conditions that may be contributing to your sciatica.

2. Physical examination

The physical exam typically includes a check of your posture, spine alignment, and reflexes. In addition, the healthcare provider will evaluate your leg muscle strength and sensation, as well as your range of motion. During this examination, the doctor may administer specific tests, such as the Straight Leg Raise Test, to help identify nerve root irritation or compression in the lower back.

3. Imaging tests

If necessary, your healthcare provider may recommend imaging studies to determine the cause of your sciatica and rule out other possibilities. Common imaging tests include the following:

- ❖ X-rays can provide an overview of the spine's bones and aid in the detection of conditions such as fractures, spinal stenosis, and bone spurs.
- ❖ MRI (Magnetic Resonance Imaging): An MRI produces detailed images of soft tissues, including the spinal discs and

nerves, which aid in the diagnosis of conditions such as herniated discs, spinal stenosis, and tumors.

❖ CT Scan (Computed Tomography): A CT scan is another imaging option that can provide a more detailed view of the spine and nerves, allowing for the detection of abnormalities that may not be visible on X-rays.

4. Nerve studies and electromyography (EMG)

In some cases, your doctor may recommend nerve conduction studies or an electromyogram (EMG) to assess how well the sciatic nerve and muscles work. These tests help to determine the extent of nerve damage, whether nerve conduction is impaired, and how the muscles respond to nerve signals.

Treatment options for sciatica

Once the cause of your sciatica has been identified, your healthcare provider will discuss treatment options. This may include:

❖ A physical therapist can lead you through exercises that will relieve pressure on the sciatic nerve, improve flexibility, and strengthen the muscles that support the spine.

❖ Medications: Over-the-counter pain relievers such as ibuprofen and acetaminophen can help reduce inflammation and pain. In some cases, your doctor may prescribe more potent medications, such as muscle relaxants, oral steroids, or nerve pain medications.

❖ Epidural Steroid Injections: If other treatments fail, your doctor may prescribe corticosteroid injections to reduce inflammation and pain in the affected area.

❖ Surgery: If conservative treatments fail to relieve severe sciatica caused by conditions such as a herniated disc or spinal stenosis, surgery may be recommended. Depending on the cause of nerve compression, surgical options include a discectomy, laminectomy, or spinal fusion.

Sciatica can be a crippling condition that disrupts a person's daily life. While mild cases may improve with conservative treatments, it is critical to seek medical attention if the pain is severe, persistent, or accompanied by other alarming symptoms such as weakness, numbness, or loss of bladder control. Early intervention and a comprehensive treatment plan tailored to the underlying cause can help relieve pain, prevent additional nerve damage, and improve overall quality of life. If you experience any of the red-flag symptoms listed above, consult a doctor to determine the best course of action.

Advantages Of Exercises For Sciatica Pain Relief

Sciatica pain, which is caused by compression or irritation of the sciatic nerve, can range from mild discomfort to debilitating pain that radiates from the lower back down the hips, buttocks, and legs. It has a significant impact on mobility, quality of life, and emotional well-being. While medication and physical therapy are frequently recommended, exercises have shown to be one of the most effective ways to manage sciatica pain. People suffering from sciatica can benefit from specific exercises that relieve pain, improve mobility, and even promote long-term recovery.

Here are some key ways that exercise helps relieve sciatica pain:

1. Strengthening core muscles to support the spine

A strong core supports the lower back and spine. When the core muscles, including the abdominal and lower back muscles, are strong, they reduce pressure on the spinal discs and vertebrae, relieving some of the pressure on the sciatic nerve. Strengthening these muscles also aids in maintaining proper posture, preventing movements and habits that may exacerbate sciatica pain.

Sciatica patients are often advised to perform core exercises like planks, partial crunches, and pelvic tilts. These exercises improve core strength, which helps stabilize the spine, prevent future injury, and reduce the risk of recurring sciatic pain.

2. Increasing flexibility and reducing muscle tension

Many cases of sciatica are associated with tight muscles in the hips, lower back, and hamstrings. Tight hamstrings, for example, can pull on the pelvis, causing tension and pain in the lower back. Similarly, tight hip flexors or piriformis muscles (a small muscle deep in the buttocks) can press on the sciatic nerve, causing or exacerbating pain.

Exercises that stretch these muscles, such as hamstring stretches, piriformis stretches, and hip flexor stretches, can help relieve muscle tension and improve flexibility. Increased flexibility reduces nerve compression, allowing for more fluid, and painless movement. Regular stretching in a sciatica management routine addresses the underlying muscle tightness and imbalance that frequently cause sciatic pain.

3. Improving blood flow and promoting healing

Exercise increases circulation, which is necessary for healing and reducing inflammation. Improved blood flow helps to deliver oxygen and nutrients to the muscles and nerves, including the sciatic nerve, assisting in their repair and reducing pain over time. Exercises that target the lower back, hips, and legs increase blood flow to these areas, which reduces inflammation that can worsen sciatica.

Gentle aerobic exercises like walking or cycling are especially good for increasing blood flow. When combined with strength and flexibility exercises, these activities stimulate the body's natural healing processes, reducing sciatica symptoms and preventing future flare-ups.

4. Reducing pain sensitivity with endorphin release

Exercise promotes the release of endorphins, the body's natural pain relievers. Endorphins interact with brain receptors to reduce pain and promote feelings of well-being. For sciatica sufferers, the increase in endorphins caused by exercise can reduce pain and improve mood, providing a natural way to cope with chronic discomfort.

Endorphin release not only makes pain management easier but also reduces the need for pain medications, which can have long-term side effects. Sciatica patients can achieve consistent pain relief without medication by incorporating regular exercise into their pain management routine.

5. Encouraging better posture and alignment

Poor posture can be both the cause and the result of sciatica. Slouching or sitting for extended periods of time can strain the lower back and cause sciatic nerve compression. Exercises that focus on core strength, flexibility, and balance can help to align the spine and pelvis, allowing for better posture during daily activities.

Good posture helps to relieve unnecessary pressure on the spine and sciatic nerve. Exercise helps to maintain a more natural alignment and prevent further aggravation of sciatica by strengthening muscle groups that support an upright posture, such as the core, lower back, and gluteal muscles.

6. Increasing stability and balance

Sciatica can impair stability, particularly if the pain or numbness spreads down the legs. Balance and stability exercises, such as standing leg lifts, side leg raises, or simple one-leg balancing, can improve coordination, strengthen supporting muscles, and lower the risk of falling or injury. Stability exercises promote the use of muscles that protect the spine and lower back, ensuring safe and controlled movements.

People with sciatica can improve their functional fitness by performing these exercises, making it easier to perform daily tasks and regain independence. Improved stability also leads to a greater sense of confidence in moving without pain.

7. Preventing muscle weakness and atrophy

Sciatica pain can discourage movement, creating a cycle of inactivity. Over time, this can lead to muscle weakness and atrophy (muscle loss), especially in the legs, glutes, and lower back. The weaker these muscles become, the less support they provide to the spine, increasing the risk of pain recurrence.

Sciatica patients can avoid muscle deterioration by staying active and focusing on targeted exercises. Consistent exercise keeps muscles active, ensuring that they remain strong and capable of supporting the spine while reducing nerve compression. This is especially important for seniors, who may already be at risk of muscle loss from aging.

8. Reduce inflammation and swelling

Sciatica is frequently accompanied by inflammation surrounding the sciatic nerve, which can exacerbate pain. Regular exercise, especially low-impact aerobic activities like swimming or walking, can help reduce inflammation. These activities improve circulation, promote muscle recovery, and reduce the body's inflammatory response.

For sciatica patients, reducing inflammation can mean the difference between constant pain and intermittent relief. Exercise reduces inflammation, providing immediate and long-term relief from sciatic pain.

9. Improving mental health and reduced stress

Living with chronic pain can hurt mental health, causing stress, anxiety, and depression. Exercise has well-documented mental health benefits, such as stress reduction and mood improvement. Physical activity causes the release of serotonin and other neurotransmitters, which improve mood, lower anxiety, and boost self-esteem.

Regular exercise not only relieves physical pain but also promotes a positive mental state. This can be extremely helpful for sciatica patients who would otherwise feel overwhelmed by their pain. A positive mental state can also help you stick to an exercise program, resulting in a cycle of improvement.

10. Promoting long-term independence and mobility

One of the most significant advantages of exercise for people with sciatica is the ability to regain mobility and independence. Consistent exercise increases the body's strength and flexibility, making everyday movements easier and less painful. Enhanced physical fitness allows sciatica patients to regain their independence, allowing them to participate in activities that they might have avoided due to pain.

Regular exercise improves quality of life by allowing people to control their pain and live an active, independent lifestyle. Sciatica patients who follow a structured exercise program can reduce their reliance on medications, avoid invasive treatments, and live a more active, pain-free life.

In conclusion, exercise has numerous benefits for managing and relieving sciatica pain, such as core strengthening, increased flexibility, improved circulation, and better posture. It also improves mental health, reduces inflammation, and fosters a sense of independence. Sciatica patients can actively participate in their healing by incorporating exercise into their daily routine, resulting in long-term pain relief and a higher quality of life.

CHAPTER 2: PREPARING FOR SCIATICA RELIEF EXERCISES

Safety Considerations For Seniors And Beginners

For seniors and beginners, beginning an exercise routine, particularly for pain relief, should always be approached with caution. Sciatica exercises can help reduce pain and improve mobility, but they must be done carefully to avoid worsening symptoms or causing new injuries. Understanding your physical limitations, choosing appropriate exercises, and maintaining a supportive environment are all important considerations.

1. Consult a healthcare professional first

Before beginning any exercise program, consult with a healthcare provider, especially if you are experiencing chronic pain or have a history of health issues. Medical advice is required to ensure that the exercises do not aggravate sciatica symptoms or interfere with any existing treatments.

2. Know your physical limitations

Seniors and beginners frequently struggle to recognize and understand their physical limitations. Sciatica often limits mobility, so start with gentle movements. Other conditions that affect a senior's exercise tolerance include arthritis and osteoporosis. Listening to your body and knowing when to stop or modify exercises is critical. It's recommended that:

- ❖ Begin with low-impact exercises.
- ❖ Avoid making sudden, jerky movements.
- ❖ Stop any movement that produces sharp or radiating pain.

3. Begin with low-impact movements

Low-impact exercises are beneficial for sciatica because they reduce stress on the joints and spine. These movements are ideal for seniors and beginners because they improve circulation, flexibility, and strength without putting too much strain on the body. Examples include seated leg lifts, gentle hamstring stretches, and slow, controlled wall push-ups. Low-impact exercises help you build strength gradually, making it easier to progress to more difficult movements over time.

4. Use the proper form and technique

Correct form is essential for avoiding injury and ensuring that the exercise targets the right muscles. Poor technique can add stress to the sciatic nerve, lower back, and other joints, potentially exacerbating symptoms. Here are some tips to maintain proper form:

- ❖ Engage the core during exercises to support the lower back.

❖ Instead of moving quickly or suddenly, keep your movements slow and controlled.
❖ If possible, use a mirror to check your posture.
❖ Seek advice from a trainer or physical therapist, especially in the beginning, to ensure proper form.

5. Warm up and cool down properly

Warming up is necessary to get the body ready for movement. A warm-up increases blood flow to the muscles, gradually loosens joints, and lowers the likelihood of strains and pulls. For beginners and seniors, a warm-up could consist of gentle stretches and light aerobic movements like arm circles or ankle rotations. Cooling down after exercise is equally important for relaxing muscles, reducing stiffness, and promoting recovery. Gentle stretching and deep breathing exercises are excellent for cooling down and reducing post-workout muscle pain.

6. Incorporate rest and recovery

Beginners and seniors may require more time to recover due to lower muscle resilience and slower healing times. Overworking the body can worsen sciatica symptoms, causing more inflammation and discomfort. Aim for moderate exercise sessions with adequate rest in between workouts, and start with a schedule that allows for two or three days of exercise per week. Gradually increasing frequency is more sustainable and reduces the risk of setbacks.

7. Maintain a safe environment

Creating a safe exercise environment is critical, particularly for seniors who are at risk of falling. Clear the workout area of any clutter, such as cords, rugs, or loose items, and make sure the floor isn't slippery. A sturdy chair or railing nearby for balance support can be beneficial for beginners who require extra stability.

8. Use supportive equipment

Supportive equipment, such as resistance bands, light hand weights, or stability balls, can help seniors and beginners perform exercises more effectively while reducing strain. A thick, nonslip mat is also useful for floor exercises. A chair with a backrest can also provide stability for certain seated exercises, making them easier to perform safely.

9. Focus on core strength and balance

Weak core muscles can put extra strain on the lower back, worsening sciatica pain. Core strengthening exercises, such as pelvic tilts or seated knee raises, help to stabilize the spine and relieve pressure on the sciatic nerve. Incorporating simple balance exercises, such as standing with one foot slightly raised, can help seniors improve stability and reduce their risk of falling. Developing core strength and balance not only alleviates sciatica but also boosts overall physical endurance.

10. Adapt exercises as needed

Adapting exercises to individual capabilities is an important safety consideration. Many exercises can be modified to reduce their range of motion or intensity, making them more suitable for people with limited flexibility or strength. For example, if standing hamstring stretches are too strenuous, try seated stretches. Beginners and seniors should avoid forcing their bodies into positions that are uncomfortable, painful, or outside of their range.

11. Practice deep breathing techniques

Incorporating breathing techniques into exercise routines can help with pain management, stress reduction, and relaxation. Deep breathing is especially beneficial for sciatica patients because it relaxes the nervous system and relieves tension in the lower back. Controlled breathing during exercise ensures that adequate oxygen flows to the muscles, reducing fatigue and maintaining energy levels.

12. Avoid excessive stretching and extreme movements

Overstretching can strain muscles and worsen sciatica pain, particularly in people who have tight lower back and leg muscles. Seniors and beginners should aim for mild to moderate stretches that don't cause pain. Extreme bending and twisting movements should also be avoided because they can compress the sciatic nerve and exacerbate symptoms. Gentle, gradual stretching is more effective and safer at relieving pain over time.

13. Set realistic goals and monitor your progress

Setting attainable goals keeps you motivated while also allowing you to track improvements in flexibility, strength, and pain levels. Beginners can set goals as small as completing one or two exercises per session and gradually increase over time. Tracking progress, such as how long you can hold a stretch or how much flexibility has improved, is both encouraging and useful for determining whether the exercise routine needs to be adjusted.

14. Be patient and consistent

For seniors and beginners, consistency is more important than intensity when managing sciatica through exercise. Results from sciatica relief exercises are often gradual, so be patient and commit to a routine without expecting immediate results.

Missing a session here and there won't hurt, but sticking to a consistent schedule will result in better, longer-term results.

15. Know when to stop

It's critical to understand when it's time to take a break or stop completely. If an exercise causes sharp, sudden pain, or if sciatica symptoms worsen after certain movements, it is best to pause and reassess. Gentle stretching and breathing exercises can provide relief without exacerbating symptoms. Always listen to your body and avoid doing exercises that don't feel right.

Exercise for sciatica relief can be safe and beneficial for both seniors and beginners if done correctly. Taking into account personal limitations, practicing proper technique, and maintaining a safe environment are all necessary steps in developing a long-term and effective exercise routine. With patience and consistency, these safety precautions can help you achieve greater strength, flexibility, and independence while relieving your pain.

Equipment Checklist: What You Need And Why

Creating a suitable environment for sciatica relief exercises entails having the proper equipment. While exercises for sciatica relief do not typically require specialized equipment, having a few basic tools can significantly improve safety, comfort, and effectiveness. *Here's a detailed look at the necessary equipment, its roles in your exercise routine, and why each piece is important for anyone, especially beginners and seniors dealing with sciatica.*

1. Exercise Mat

An exercise mat is a cushioned, non-slip surface that allows you to safely perform stretches, core work, and strengthening exercises. Sciatica exercises frequently include movements that require lying, kneeling, or sitting on the ground. A quality mat cushions sensitive joints such as the knees, hips, and back, reducing discomfort and the risk of injury from hard surfaces. Furthermore, the nonslip material keeps the mat from moving, which aids in stability during standing or balance exercises.

2. Supportive Chair with a Stable Base

A sturdy chair provides stable support for both seated and standing exercises. Many sciatica relief exercises for seniors include modifications that can be performed seated or with chair support. Stretches such as the seated spinal twist and standing balance exercises, for example, can be done safely with the help of a stable chair. Look for a chair with no wheels and, ideally, a backrest to provide extra support. This reduces strain on the lower back and provides a safe and easy way to improve flexibility and strength.

3. Resistance Bands

Resistance bands are lightweight, stretchy bands that provide gentle resistance during exercises. Resistance bands can help strengthen the muscles in your lower back, core, and legs, which are essential for sciatica relief. Resistance bands come in a variety of tension levels, making them a versatile tool for gradually increasing the challenge as you build strength. They are also extremely portable, making them ideal for home workouts or use on the go. To strengthen key muscle groups, use a resistance band with exercises such as leg raises, hip abductions, and side-lying clamshells.

4. Foam Rollers or Massage Balls

Foam rollers and massage balls are self-massage tools that aid in muscle relaxation and blood circulation. Foam rolling or using a massage ball can help release tight muscles and fascia that can cause sciatica pain. Tight muscles in the glutes, hamstrings, and lower back can put pressure on the sciatic nerve. Rolling over these areas can help reduce muscle tension and increase flexibility, thereby alleviating sciatica symptoms. Foam rollers are excellent for larger muscles, whereas massage balls are ideal for smaller, more specific areas such as the glutes or piriformis muscle, which is a common cause of sciatica pain.

5. Yoga Blocks

Yoga blocks add support and height to certain poses and stretches, making them more accessible. Yoga blocks can be extremely beneficial to people with limited flexibility or mobility. They allow you to stretch comfortably, reducing the risk of overstretching or straining. For example, in hamstring stretches, place blocks under your hands to support your torso, reducing strain on your lower back. They're also great for seated poses, as they raise the hips and relieve pressure on the sciatic nerve.

6. Stretching or Yoga Strap

A stretching or yoga strap can help you reach or hold stretches, especially if you have limited flexibility. A strap can help you safely extend your range in different stretches without putting too much strain on your lower back. It's useful for hamstring stretches, for example, by looping the strap around the foot and gently pulling to deepen the stretch. This helps relieve hamstring tightness, which, if left untreated, can exacerbate sciatica symptoms.

7. A Small Stability Ball or Pilates ball

A small stability ball, usually 9-12 inches in diameter, is used to engage core muscles and aid in gentle strength exercises. Stability balls provide a unique way to gently and safely activate core muscles, which is essential for spinal support and sciatica pain relief. For example, while seated, place a small stability ball behind your lower back to help support and engage your core during exercises. They're also great for knee squeezes and pelvic tilts, which work the muscles in your lower back and hips.

8. Towel or Cushion

Towels and cushions are simple props that can provide comfort or support while exercising. Towels and cushions can be used to provide extra padding, particularly for seniors who may be experiencing knee, hip, or lower back discomfort. For example, placing a folded towel under your knees during certain stretches or under your back for extra lumbar support can make exercises more comfortable and less stressful in sensitive areas. They can also be used to provide gentle support during seated exercises, or as a small resistance tool by squeezing a rolled-up towel between your knees.

9. Mirror

A mirror helps you check and adjust your form while exercising. Why It's Important: Proper form is essential for beginners, seniors, and anyone new to specific exercises to avoid injury and ensure that each movement is effective. A mirror provides instant feedback on posture, alignment, and body position. For example, a mirror can help you avoid straining your back or misaligning your body while performing exercises like planks or wall squats.

10. Comfortable and Supportive Footwear

Proper footwear provides a stable base for standing exercises, lowering the risk of slipping and falling. Stretches and movements involving weight shifting and balance are frequently used in sciatica relief exercises. Supportive shoes with non-slip soles reduce the risk of injury and provide extra support for the feet, ankles, and lower body. Proper footwear can also relieve pressure on the lower back and legs, thereby reducing sciatic pain.

Bonus: Optional Equipment

- ❖ *Ankle Weights:* After gaining strength, ankle weights can be used to gradually increase the difficulty of leg exercises.
- ❖ *Portable Workout Bar or Rail:* A secure bar or rail can provide support for balance exercises, particularly for those working on stability.
- ❖ *Timer or Stopwatch:* Tracking exercise duration and rest times allows you to maintain consistency while gradually increasing endurance.

The right equipment does more than just make exercises easier; it improves safety, reduces discomfort, and allows you to make the most of each movement. Each piece of equipment on this checklist contributes uniquely to the development of strength, flexibility, and stability, all of which are necessary for sciatica management and regaining independence.

Tips for Selecting Quality Equipment

A comfortable and effective sciatica exercise routine requires the use of high-quality equipment. Here are some useful tips to help you choose the right items for long-term use while ensuring safety, durability, and ease of use:

1. Prioritize durability

Long-lasting equipment saves money and provides stability, particularly for seniors and beginners who require consistent support. Choose items made of high-quality materials, such as thick foam mats, heavy-duty resistance bands, and durable chairs. Avoid flimsy options that will wear out quickly or break under pressure.

2. Choose non-slip surfaces

Non-slip surfaces are essential for stability, particularly in exercises that require stretching, balance, or weight shifting. Non-slip textures or coatings on mats and other equipment help to prevent slipping and increase safety. Non-slip features are especially useful for stability exercises or for those who are just getting started and require extra grip.

3. Ensure comfort and ergonomic design

Comfortable, well-designed equipment can relieve strain on sensitive areas such as the lower back and knees, allowing you to exercise more easily. Select items with comfort features, such as cushioned mats or foam-covered handles on resistance bands. Choose chairs with comfortable seats and backrests to support the body while exercising.

4. Select portable and space-saving options

Compact, portable equipment makes it simple to maintain a home routine, especially when working with limited space. Folding chairs, small stability balls, and resistance bands are all lightweight and easy to store. Consider collapsible or compact designs that allow you to store equipment easily without cluttering up your space.

5. Check for adjustability and versatility

Adjustable equipment can be tailored to various fitness levels and body types, allowing you to progress safely. Some resistance bands come in sets with varying tension levels that can be switched out as your strength grows. Yoga blocks, for example, come in a variety of sizes and can be stacked for additional support.

6. Look for easy maintenance

Equipment that is simple to clean and maintain will last longer and help you maintain a sanitary workout space. Choose washable or easy-to-clean mats, especially if they will be used on bare skin. Look for foam rollers and resistance bands that are water-resistant or coated so they can be cleaned regularly.

7. Check for smooth functionality

Well-functioning equipment enables safe, controlled movements, which are critical for relieving sciatica pain without strain or injury. Ensure that resistance bands stretch evenly without snapping or catching and that foam rollers are firm but not overly rigid. If possible, try items in-store to ensure smoothness and ease of use.

8. Consider weight and mobility

Lightweight equipment is easier to handle, especially for seniors who may require assistance moving items or arranging their workout space. Lightweight yoga blocks, small stability balls, and resistance bands that are easy to transport. Avoid items that are extremely heavy and may be difficult to lift or transport safely.

9. Seek high-quality support features

Quality support features improve comfort and stability, especially in chairs and mats. Chairs should be sturdy and have a strong backrest. Check the thickness and density of mats; a thicker mat provides better cushioning for joints while remaining firm enough to maintain stability during exercises.

10. Evaluate product warranties and customer feedback

Warranties and customer reviews provide information about the product's durability and quality. Look for brands that provide warranties or guarantees, as this often indicates the manufacturer's confidence in their product. Additionally, read customer reviews to learn from others' experiences and identify any common issues.

By carefully considering these tips when purchasing equipment, you will be better prepared to select items that are appropriate for your fitness level, physical needs, and workout space. Having the right tools helps to create a supportive, comfortable environment, which makes it easier to stick with your sciatica relief exercises over time.

Tips For Creating A Comfortable Workout Space At Home

Creating a comfortable workout space at home is essential for keeping your exercise routine safe, motivating, and enjoyable. For people suffering from conditions such as sciatica or mobility issues, having a well-prepared space can improve both effectiveness and safety. *Here are some important tips to consider when setting up your home workout area:*

1. Choose the right location

Choose a location in your home where you can exercise without interruption. A designated area allows you to store necessary equipment while also developing the habit of using the space regularly. This could be a spare room, a corner of the living room, or even a section of the garage.

Make sure the area is large enough to accommodate all of the exercises in your routine. To avoid injury, make sure you have enough room to stretch your arms, lie down, and extend your legs without hitting any walls or furniture. If possible, choose a room with windows to allow for natural light and fresh air. Good lighting improves mood, and fresh air keeps the room from feeling stuffy. If windows are not available, consider using bright artificial lighting and an air purifier or fan to circulate the air.

2. Create a comfortable flooring surface

Safety is critical, especially for seniors and beginners who may have balance issues. Choose flooring with a stable, nonslip surface. Hardwood, rubber flooring, and exercise mats are all good options. If your floor is hard, use exercise mats to provide extra cushioning, especially for exercises that require lying or sitting on the floor. Mats with extra padding can also protect your knees, hips, and spine while exercising, reducing impact and discomfort.

If you have rugs or carpets in your workout area, make sure they do not slip. Non-slip pads or adhesive strips beneath rugs can help keep them in place and prevent accidental slips while moving.

3. Organize essential equipment for convenience

Keeping your setup simple with only the necessities can help it feel less cluttered and more functional. A sciatica workout may require resistance bands, dumbbells, a chair for support, and a yoga mat. Storage solutions, such as shelves, baskets, or cabinets, can help keep equipment organized and out of the way when not in use. Consider using a small weight rack or a basket to store resistance bands and mats.

Items such as foam rollers, straps, or cushions should be easily accessible, especially if you need them during an exercise. Having these within arm's reach allows your workout to continue uninterrupted and reduces strain from bending or reaching.

4. Prioritize safety and accessibility

Make sure there are no sharp edges, furniture corners, or low-hanging decorations that could interfere with movement. Declutter the area so you can move freely while reducing the risk of tripping. For balance and safety, keep a sturdy chair or wall nearby to use if you feel unsteady. This is especially useful for seniors and beginners because it boosts confidence and support during balance exercises.

When performing exercises that require lying down or floor work, using thick mats or placing extra cushions nearby can provide additional protection and comfort.

5. Optimize lighting and temperature

Adequate lighting is required not only for safety but also to maintain an energetic environment. Natural light is preferable, but if that isn't possible, use bright LED lighting. Adjust the lighting to avoid shadows, which can make the space appear cramped or uninviting. Working out at the proper temperature helps to avoid discomfort and overheating. Keep a fan, air conditioner, or space heater on hand to keep the temperature comfortable during your workout.

Mirrors can help beginners check their forms and ensure that exercises are performed safely and correctly. A full-length mirror placed where you can see your movements can improve alignment and confidence.

6. Create an inviting and calming atmosphere

Motivational quotes, a vision board, or photos of places you enjoy can help you stay motivated and focused on your goals. Adding a few plants can help purify the air while also creating a calm, natural atmosphere. This is especially comforting if your exercises are centered on relaxation and pain relief. If you enjoy certain scents, try using a diffuser with essential oils such as lavender or eucalyptus. Aromatherapy can help you relax and develop a positive association with your workout space.

7. Set up a device for guided workouts and music

If you use guided workouts or video tutorials, place a tablet, laptop, or TV where you can easily see them. Position it at eye level to avoid straining your neck while exercising. Music can increase energy and make exercise more enjoyable. Consider putting a small speaker in your workout area or wearing headphones if you're in a shared space. Music with a steady beat is ideal for keeping pace, whereas relaxing music can help with slower, more focused stretches.

8. Plan for your post-workout needs

Staying hydrated requires keeping a water bottle within reach. A towel can also be useful for removing sweat during or after a workout. Set aside a small area with a foam roller, stretching strap, or even a comfortable chair to cool down and stretch after your workout. This area can be used for gentle relaxation exercises that benefit both the body and mind. For those suffering from chronic pain, keeping an ice pack or heating pad on hand can provide immediate relief if discomfort arises during the session.

9. Adjust the layout as necessary for flexibility

As you become more accustomed to your workout routine, you may want to change the layout. If you add new exercises or equipment, make sure your setup allows for smooth transitions between activities. Depending on the season, you may require more or less airflow and lighting. Adjust fans, heaters, and curtains as needed to keep your workout area comfortable year-round.

10. Establish boundaries for focus and privacy

If you live with others, discuss your workout schedule and request uninterrupted time in the space. This allows you to stay focused and completely engaged in your routine. If your workout area is part of a shared space, consider using visual dividers such as a folding screen or an area rug to mark the workout zone. This helps to mentally separate your exercise space from the rest of your home, making it feel more dedicated and purposeful.

Setting up a dedicated, comfortable, and practical workout space at home creates an environment that promotes your health journey. The right setup not only makes it easier to stick to your routine but also ensures that each workout is safe and fun.

CHAPTER 3: GENTLE WARM-UP EXERCISES FOR SAFE MOVEMENT

The Significance Of Warming Up To Prevent Harm

Warming up is an important part of any exercise routine and can help prevent injuries, especially for people who have pre-existing conditions or are starting a new workout regimen. When done correctly, a warm-up session prepares the body for more intense activity, lowers the risk of strain, and improves overall performance. A warm-up routine is essential for individuals with conditions such as sciatica, as well as those who are older and may be more prone to injury.

What is a Warm-up?

A warm-up is a low-intensity, preparatory phase that occurs before beginning the main exercise or workout routine. It typically consists of gentle movements, dynamic stretching, and breathing exercises designed to gradually increase heart rate, blood flow, and joint mobility. Warm-ups are intended to gradually and systematically prepare the body for more strenuous physical activity, allowing muscles, tendons, and joints to adapt and prepare for the challenges ahead. A good warm-up can last anywhere from 5 to 15 minutes, depending on the individual's needs, fitness level, and subsequent exercise.

Physiological Benefits of Warming Up

1. **Improves blood flow and oxygen supply:** When you begin a warm-up routine, your heart rate rises, which increases blood flow to the muscles. This increased blood circulation ensures that more oxygen reaches muscle tissues. More oxygen primes muscles to handle greater exertion, lowering the likelihood of strains or injuries. For example, dynamic movements such as arm circles, leg swings, and gentle marches gradually raise the heart rate, improving blood circulation without putting undue strain on the body.

2. **Raises muscle temperature:** Warming up also raises muscle temperature, which improves performance and helps to prevent injuries. Warmer muscles are more elastic and less prone to tears or strains during stretching and strength training. When the muscle temperature rises, the elasticity of muscle fibers increases, allowing them to stretch and contract more effectively. This increased flexibility reduces the risk of injury to tendons and ligaments because they can better respond to sudden or intense movements.

3. **Enhances synovial fluid production:** Joint mobility is another important factor in avoiding injuries. During a warm-up, the body produces more synovial fluid, which lubricates joints and reduces friction between bones. This lubrication allows the joints to move more smoothly and

reduces the risk of joint injuries, particularly during exercises that require bending, twisting, or lifting. For those suffering from sciatica or lower back pain, a well-lubricated joint system allows for greater mobility and less discomfort.

Neuromuscular Benefits of Warming Up

1. **Enhances muscle coordination and activation:** A warm-up session activates the muscles that will be used in the upcoming workout, allowing them to fully engage and function as a unit. When muscles are activated, they can better coordinate their movements, which is especially beneficial in exercises that require balance, stability, and control. Warm-up exercises frequently include dynamic stretches that mimic the primary workout movements but at a slower pace, allowing the nervous system to become acquainted with the movements and improving muscle memory.

2. **Prepares the nervous system:** The nervous system has an important role in movement coordination and response. Warming up gradually stimulates the nervous system, allowing the brain and muscles to communicate more effectively. This stimulation improves reflexes, balance, and reaction times, all of which are necessary to avoid missteps, falls, or unexpected twists that could cause injury. Warming up also allows the brain to mentally prepare for the demands

of exercise, which aids in focusing attention on correct form and technique.

Psychological Benefits of Warming Up

1. **Improves mental focus and preparedness:** A warm-up focuses not only on physical preparation but also on mental readiness. Warming up allows you to focus on the upcoming workout, clear your mind, and fully engage in each movement. This level of concentration is especially beneficial for beginners and people suffering from chronic pain, as it helps them gain confidence and awareness of their bodies.

2. **Reduces anxiety and increases confidence:** A warm-up can help people who are new to exercise or who are recovering from an injury feel more in control and familiar with their surroundings. Starting with gentle, low-impact movements reduces anxiety about physical activity and boosts confidence in one's ability to complete the exercises without causing pain or re-injury. Individuals feel more confident in attempting the main exercises when their muscles are prepared and movements are practiced at a slower pace.

Warming up is not an optional step, but rather an essential component of safe and effective exercise. It physically prepares the body by increasing circulation, raising muscle temperature, and activating the nervous system, while also providing psychological benefits such as increased focus and confidence. For beginners, seniors, and people suffering from sciatica, a warm-up can mean the difference between a successful, pain-relieving workout and a dangerous one. Whether it's a simple stretching session or a light cardio routine, warm-ups are critical for avoiding injury and getting the most out of each exercise session.

Consequences Of Skipping Warm-Up

Skipping a warm-up can cause a variety of physical and performance issues. Here are some of the primary consequences that may result from jumping right into an exercise routine without adequate preparation:

1. Higher risk of muscle strains and tears: Cold muscles lack the elasticity and flexibility of warmed-up muscles, making them more susceptible to unexpected tears or strains. Muscles become stiff and easily overextended without a warm-up, particularly during intense or fast-paced movements.

2. Increased risk of joint injuries: Joints require lubrication to move smoothly, which is accomplished by increasing synovial fluid production during a warm-up. Without this, joints can stiffen, increasing the likelihood of sprains, particularly in the knees, hips, and ankles. Joint injuries can be especially difficult for seniors or those with conditions such as sciatica, as recovery may take longer and cause additional mobility issues.

3. Reduced range of motion and flexibility: A warm-up relaxes muscles and ligaments, increasing flexibility and range of motion. Without it, the body may feel tight, limiting

performance, reducing movement efficiency, and raising the risk of overstretching or straining.

4. Poorer coordination and balance: The nervous system is essential for coordinating movements. A warm-up stimulates this system, improving muscle coordination and reaction time. Skipping this step can result in decreased balance and control, which can lead to unintentional missteps, slips, or falls—especially dangerous for beginners and seniors.

5. Reduced endurance and early fatigue: Warming up prepares muscles for efficient energy production, which is required to maintain endurance during exercise. Skipping this step can cause premature fatigue, making the workout feel more strenuous than necessary and potentially shortening it.

6. Increased heart and respiratory rates: A warm-up gradually raises heart rate and primes the cardiovascular system for exercise. Without this preparation, a person may experience sudden, uncomfortable spikes in heart rate or breathing, which can cause dizziness, shortness of breath, and, in some cases, heart strain.

7. Delayed recovery and increased soreness: Warming up reduces the buildup of lactic acid in muscles by gradually preparing the body for physical activity. Without it, muscles are more likely to feel sore and stiff after exercise, resulting

in longer recovery times and discomfort, particularly for those with muscle-related conditions.

8. Mental unpreparedness and decreased focus: Skipping the warm-up has an impact on mental readiness. A proper warm-up improves mental focus, establishes proper form, and boosts confidence for the upcoming workout. Without this, it's easy to feel rushed, unfocused, or distracted, increasing the likelihood of using poor technique and risking further injury.

Skipping a warm-up can increase the risk of injury, discomfort, and even poor performance. Taking the time to properly warm up ensures a safer, more effective workout with improved results and long-term health benefits.

Simple Warm-Up Routines To Loosen Tight Muscles

1. Marching in Place (2–3 Minutes)

Marching in place is an easy way to increase your heart rate and get blood flowing throughout the body.

1. Stand tall with your feet hip-width apart.
2. Lift one knee to hip level, then switch to the other leg in a marching motion.
3. Swing your arms naturally with each march.
4. Continue for 2–3 minutes, focusing on smooth, controlled movements.

2. Arm Circles (1–2 Minutes)

Arm circles help loosen the shoulders, upper back, and neck muscles.

1. Extend your arms out to your sides at shoulder height.
2. Start making small circles with your arms, gradually increasing the size of the circles.
3. Do this for about 30 seconds in one direction, then switch directions.
4. Repeat twice for each direction.

3. Cat-Cow Stretch (1–2 Minutes)

This gentle stretch, often used in yoga, helps to mobilize the spine and loosen the lower back muscles.

1. Start on all fours, with your wrists under your shoulders and knees under your hips.
2. Inhale as you arch your back, dropping your belly toward the floor and lifting your chest and tailbone (Cow Pose).
3. Exhale as you round your spine, tucking your chin to your chest and drawing your belly button toward your spine (Cat Pose).
4. Continue moving between Cat and Cow for 1–2 minutes, moving slowly with each breath.

4. Leg Swings (1–2 Minutes)

Leg swings help loosen the hip flexors, hamstrings, and lower back.

1. Stand next to a wall or a chair for support.
2. Swing one leg forward and backward in a controlled motion, keeping your upper body stable.
3. Do 10–15 swings on each leg.
4. Then, turn to face the wall or chair and swing each leg side to side for 10–15 swings per leg.

5. Shoulder Shrugs (1–2 Minutes)

Shoulder shrugs relieve tension in the shoulders and neck.

1. Stand or sit comfortably with your arms relaxed at your sides.
2. Inhale deeply as you lift both shoulders toward your ears.
3. Exhale as you release your shoulders back down.
4. Repeat for 1–2 minutes, keeping the motion slow and controlled.

6. Gentle Torso Twists (1–2 Minutes)

Torso twists loosen up the lower back and sides, preparing the core for movement.

1. Stand with your feet hip-width apart and hands on your hips.
2. Slowly twist your torso to the right, then to the left.
3. Keep your hips facing forward and twist from the waist.
4. Perform 10–15 twists on each side.

7. Ankle Circles (1–2 Minutes)

Ankle circles are great for warming up the ankles and calves, especially useful before exercises that involve standing or balance.

1. Sit or stand and lift one foot slightly off the ground.
2. Slowly rotate your ankle clockwise for 10–15 circles.
3. Switch directions and do 10–15 circles counterclockwise.
4. Repeat on the other foot.

8. Knee to Chest Stretch (1–2 Minutes)

This gentle stretch releases tightness in the lower back, glutes, and hips.

1. Lie on your back with your legs extended.
2. Slowly bring one knee up toward your chest, clasping it with both hands.
3. Hold the stretch for 15–20 seconds, then switch to the other leg.
4. Repeat 2–3 times on each side.

9. Pelvic Tilts (1–2 Minutes)

Pelvic tilts help activate the core and stretch the lower back, making them excellent for sciatica relief.

1. Lie on your back with your knees bent and feet flat on the floor.
2. Slowly press your lower back into the floor by tilting your pelvis upward.
3. Hold for a few seconds, then release.
4. Repeat this motion 10–15 times, moving slowly.

10. Side Stretches (1–2 Minutes)

Side stretches help to open up the sides of the body, stretching the obliques and loosening up the rib cage.

1. Stand with your feet hip-width apart and arms at your sides.
2. Reach one arm up and over to the opposite side, bending gently at the waist.
3. Hold for a few seconds, then switch to the other side.
4. Repeat 10–15 times on each side.

Each of these warm-up exercises is designed to target different muscle groups, improve joint mobility, and increase circulation, helping to prepare the body for movement and reduce the risk of injury.

CHAPTER 4: SIMPLE SCIATICA RELIEF EXERCISES

Before you begin any sciatica cure exercises, take a minute to check in with yourself and assess your condition. Sciatica is a complex ailment that varies greatly from person to person, with symptoms ranging from minor discomfort to severe agony. Understanding your own body's limitations is critical. If you feel extreme discomfort, numbness, or weakness, it may indicate that your problem necessitates a more individualized treatment or medical intervention. Taking notes on your symptoms, their intensity, and any triggers might help you better convey your needs to a healthcare expert.

Before beginning any sciatica workout plan, consult with a healthcare specialist, such as a physical therapist, chiropractor, or doctor. A consultant can evaluate your specific case, identify the underlying reasons for your sciatica, and provide a personalized plan to effectively address your symptoms. While many basic exercises are beneficial to most people, some motions may not be suited for specific types of sciatica, such as those caused by herniated discs, spinal stenosis, or piriformis syndrome. A healthcare expert can guarantee that the workouts you're undertaking don't worsen your condition and can help you prevent damage.

A personalized approach to sciatica alleviation will examine not only the exact muscles and locations causing your pain, but also your overall health, mobility, and fitness levels. Seniors and people with other health conditions, for example, may need to modify workouts or have extra help to accomplish particular activities safely. In contrast, younger or more physically active people may benefit from more vigorous activities. Working with a professional ensures that your activities are tailored to your specific healing needs and that you are not causing more harm than good. Furthermore, a consultant may advise you on when to continue more complex workouts and when to rest, ensuring a consistent recovery with no setbacks.

1. Planks

Instructions:

1. Begin by lying face down with your forearms flat on the floor and elbows directly under your shoulders.
2. Lift your body, keeping your body in a straight line from your head to your heels.
3. Engage your core and avoid letting your hips sag or rise.
4. Hold this position for as long as you can, aiming for 20 to 30 seconds, and gradually increase the time.
5. Keep your breathing steady and controlled throughout the hold.

2. Standing Calf Raises

Instructions:

1. Stand with your feet hip-width apart, ensuring you are on a flat, firm surface.
2. Slowly raise your heels as high as you can, balancing on the balls of your feet.
3. Hold for a moment at the top, then lower back down slowly.
4. Perform 10-15 repetitions, and repeat for 2-3 sets.

3. Hip Abduction

Instructions:

1. Stand straight with a wall or chair for support.
2. Lift one leg out to the side, keeping it straight and maintaining good posture.
3. Hold for a second, then return the leg to the starting position.
4. Perform 10-15 reps on each leg, aiming for 2-3 sets.

4. Clamshell Exercise

Instructions:

1. Lie on your side with your knees bent at a 90-degree angle and feet stacked.
2. Keep your pelvis steady as you lift the top knee while keeping your feet together.
3. Pause at the top, then slowly lower the knee back down.
4. Perform 10-15 reps on each side, completing 2-3 sets.

5. Heel Slides

Instructions:

1. Lie flat on your back with your knees bent and feet flat on the floor.
2. Slowly slide one heel away from your body, straightening the leg as much as you can.
3. Slide the heel back to the starting position.
4. Alternate legs and complete 10-15 reps for each leg, performing 2-3 sets.

6. Seated Spinal Twist

Instructions:

1. Sit on a chair with your feet flat on the floor and your back straight.
2. Twist your torso to one side, reaching the opposite hand to the back of the chair.
3. Hold the position for 15-30 seconds, then switch sides.
4. Repeat 2-3 times per side.

7. Knee to Opposite Shoulder

Instructions:

1. Lie on your back with your knees bent and feet flat on the floor.
2. Bring one knee toward the opposite shoulder, holding it with both hands.
3. Hold the stretch for 15-30 seconds, then return to the starting position.
4. Repeat 2-3 times per side.

8. Stand on One Leg

Instructions:

1. Stand tall and shift your weight onto one leg.
2. Lift the other leg off the ground and hold the position for 20-30 seconds.
3. Focus on keeping your body steady and balanced.
4. Repeat 2-3 times for each leg.

9. Hamstring Curls

Instructions:

1. Stand straight with your feet hip-width apart, holding onto a sturdy chair for balance.
2. Slowly bend one knee, bringing your heel toward your glutes.
3. Hold for a second, then lower the leg back down.
4. Perform 10-15 reps on each leg, repeating for 2-3 sets.

10. Wall Pushups

Instructions:

1. Stand a few feet away from a wall and place your hands on it at shoulder height.
2. Lower your body toward the wall by bending your elbows, keeping your body in a straight line.
3. Push back to the starting position, straightening your arms.
4. Perform 10-15 reps, completing 2-3 sets.

11. Side Planks

Instructions:

1. Lie on your side with your forearm on the floor and elbow directly under your shoulder.
2. Lift your hips off the floor, forming a straight line from head to heels.
3. Hold the position for 15-30 seconds, then switch sides.
4. Repeat 2-3 times per side.

12. Quadriceps Stretch

Instructions:

1. Stand straight and grab your ankle behind you, pulling your heel toward your glutes.
2. Keep your knees close together and avoid arching your back.
3. Hold the stretch for 15-30 seconds, then repeat on the other side.
4. Perform 2-3 sets per leg.

13. Lower Back Stretches

Instructions:

1. Lie on your back with your knees bent and feet flat on the floor.
2. Slowly pull both knees toward your chest, holding them with your hands.
3. Hold for 15-30 seconds, then release.
4. Repeat 2-3 times.

14. Standing Hamstring Stretch

Instructions:

1. Stand tall with one leg extended in front of you and your heel on the ground.
2. Slowly lean forward from your hips while keeping your back straight.
3. Hold the stretch for 15-30 seconds, then switch legs.
4. Repeat 2-3 times per leg.

15. Prone Press Ups

Instructions:

1. Lie on your stomach with your hands placed flat on the floor under your shoulders.
2. Push up with your arms, arching your back slightly while keeping your hips on the floor.
3. Hold the position for a few seconds, then lower back down.
4. Perform 10-15 repetitions, completing 2-3 sets.

16. Bridge Exercise

Instructions:

1. Lie on your back with your knees bent and feet flat on the floor, hip-width apart.
2. Press through your heels and lift your hips toward the ceiling, forming a straight line from your shoulders to your knees.
3. Hold for 1-2 seconds at the top, then slowly lower your hips back down.
4. Repeat for 10-15 reps, completing 2-3 sets.

17. Wall Squats

Instructions:

1. Stand with your back against a wall and your feet a few inches in front of you.
2. Slowly slide your back down the wall, bending your knees to form a 90-degree angle.
3. Hold the squat for 10-30 seconds, then slowly rise back to standing.
4. Perform 10-15 reps for 2-3 sets.

18. Straight Leg Raises

Instructions:

1. Lie flat on your back with your legs extended and your arms by your sides.
2. Slowly lift one leg straight up, keeping it engaged and avoiding arching your back.
3. Hold for a second at the top, then lower the leg back down.
4. Perform 10-15 reps for each leg, repeating for 2-3 sets.

19. Gluteal Stretches

Instructions:

1. Lie on your back with your knees bent and feet flat on the floor.
2. Cross one ankle over the opposite knee to form a figure-four shape.
3. Gently pull the uncrossed leg toward your chest to stretch the glutes.
4. Hold for 15-30 seconds, then switch sides.
5. Repeat 2-3 times per side.

20. Cat-Cow Pose

Instructions:

1. Start on all fours with your hands directly under your shoulders and knees under your hips.
2. Inhale and arch your back (cow pose), lifting your tailbone and looking up.
3. Exhale and round your back (cat pose), tucking your chin and tailbone.
4. Repeat for 10-15 rounds, flowing smoothly between poses.

21. Piriformis Stretch

Instructions:

1. Lie on your back with your knees bent and feet flat on the floor.
2. Cross one leg over the other, placing your ankle on the opposite knee.
3. Gently pull the uncrossed leg toward your chest to stretch the piriformis muscle.
4. Hold for 15-30 seconds, then switch sides.
5. Perform 2-3 repetitions per side.

22. Lying Hamstring Stretch

Instructions:

1. Lie flat on your back with one leg extended and the other bent.
2. Hold the extended leg behind the thigh or calf and gently pull it toward you to stretch the hamstring.
3. Hold for 15-30 seconds, then switch legs.
4. Repeat 2-3 times per leg.

23. Inner Thigh Stretch

Instructions:

1. Sit on the floor with your legs spread wide apart.
2. Lean forward from your hips while keeping your back straight.
3. Reach your hands toward the floor or your feet for a deeper stretch.
4. Hold the position for 15-30 seconds, then relax.
5. Repeat 2-3 times.

24. Front Thigh Stretch

Instructions:

1. Stand tall and grab your ankle behind you, pulling your heel toward your glutes.
2. Keep your knees together and your hips aligned.
3. Hold for 15-30 seconds, then switch legs.
4. Repeat 2-3 sets per leg.

25. Calf Stretch

Instructions:

1. Stand facing a wall, placing your hands on it for support.
2. Step one leg back, keeping it straight, and press your heel into the floor.
3. Hold the stretch for 15-30 seconds, then switch legs.
4. Perform 2-3 repetitions per leg.

26. Lower Back Rotation

Instructions:

1. Lie on your back with your knees bent and feet flat on the floor.
2. Slowly drop both knees to one side, keeping your shoulders on the floor.
3. Hold for 15-30 seconds, then switch sides.
4. Repeat 2-3 times per side.

27. Child's Pose

Instructions:

1. Start on your hands and knees, then sit back on your heels with your arms extended forward.
2. Lower your forehead to the floor and relax into the stretch.
3. Hold for 30 seconds to 1 minute, focusing on deep breathing.
4. Repeat as needed.

CHAPTER 5: RELAXATION AND BREATHING TECHNIQUES FOR PAIN MANAGEMENT

Techniques For Relaxing The Nervous System And Lowering Muscle Tension

Managing muscle tension and soothing the nervous system is critical for overall health, especially for anyone suffering from sciatica, stress, or chronic pain. The body's response to stress, injury, or discomfort frequently results in tight muscles, which can aggravate pain and impede healing. Individuals who learn strategies to minimize muscle tension and soothe the nervous system can improve their quality of life, better manage pain, and promote greater relaxation. Here are numerous established approaches for accomplishing this:

1. Deep Breathing Exercises

Deep breathing exercises are one of the most powerful ways to relax the neurological system, relieve muscle tension, and manage stress. Individuals who practice controlled, steady breathing can engage the parasympathetic nerve system—the body's natural "rest and digest" system—which counteracts the "fight or flight" reaction triggered by stress. This process slows the heart rate, decreases blood pressure, and promotes relaxation, which helps to relieve both physical and mental stress. The following is an expanded guide to deep breathing exercises, including multiple techniques, advantages, and best practices for incorporating them into daily life.

Before delving into specific strategies, it's important to grasp the fundamental physiology of breathing. When we breathe, oxygen enters the lungs and is exchanged for carbon dioxide in the circulation. Shallow, fast breathing, which is prevalent under stressful or painful situations, is frequently related to sympathetic nervous system activation. Deep, leisurely breathing, on the other hand, stimulates the parasympathetic nervous system, resulting in relaxation and reduced muscle tension.

Breathing deeply from the diaphragm, as opposed to shallow chest breathing, ensures that the lungs are filled, enhancing oxygen intake and promoting nervous system relaxation.

A. Diaphragmatic Respiration (belly breathing)

Diaphragmatic breathing is the foundation of deepest breathing techniques. To fully engage the diaphragm, breathe deeply into the belly instead of the chest. This practice promotes deep relaxation and is very helpful in reducing anxiety, and tension, and boosting the body's overall ability to relax.

Instructions:

1. Find a comfortable position, whether sitting or lying down.
   If you're lying down, put a pillow beneath your head and
   knees for added support.
2. Hold one hand on your chest and the other on your abdomen
   (just below the rib cage).
3. Inhale deeply through your nose, allowing your diaphragm
   to expand and push your abdomen out. The hand on your
   abdomen should rise as you inhale, but the hand on your
   chest should stay relatively static.
4. Hold your breath for 2–4 seconds.
5. Exhale softly through your lips, releasing any tension. As
   the air exits your lungs, let your hand descend to your
   abdomen.
6. Repeat the technique for 5-10 minutes, concentrating on the
   gradual rise and fall of your abdomen with each breath.

Benefits:

1. It activates the parasympathetic nervous system, which
   promotes relaxation.
2. Reduces muscle tension by increasing oxygen delivery to the
   muscles.
3. Encourages conscious breathing, which helps with attention
   and concentration.

B. Box Breathing (square breathing)

Box breathing is a structured breathing method commonly used to alleviate anxiety and tension. It consists of breathing, holding the breath, exhaling, and holding again in equal time intervals, forming a "box" pattern. This approach promotes a rhythmic and relaxing influence on the body and mind, which is especially beneficial in stressful situations.

Instructions:

1. Sit or lie down in a comfortable position, spine straight.
2. Inhale deeply through your nose for four seconds.
3. Hold your breath for four seconds.
4. Exhale slowly and thoroughly through your mouth for a count of four seconds.
5. Hold your breath for 4 seconds before taking the next inhale.
6. Repeat the technique for 5-10 minutes.

Benefits:

1. Reduces tension by focusing the mind on the breath and keeping a consistent rhythm.
2. Helps to reduce the heart rate and blood pressure.
3. Calms the neurological system and promotes profound relaxation.

C. 4-7-8 Breathing Technique

The 4-7-8 breathing technique is a simple yet effective way to promote calm and improve sleep. By focusing on the timing of your breath, you may instantly reduce stress and help your body relax. It is especially effective when you're anxious, agitated, or trying to fall asleep.

Instructions:

1. Sit or lie down in a comfortable position, with your back straight.
2. Close your eyes and exhale entirely through your mouth, producing a whooshing sound.
3. Inhale quietly via your nose for four seconds.
4. Hold your breath for seven seconds.
5. Exhale gently through your lips for 8 seconds, generating a whooshing sound as you do.
6. Repeat the cycle 4–8 times, concentrating on the rhythm of your breath.

Benefits:

1. Encourages deeper, slower breathing, promoting a sense of peace and relaxation.
2. Reduces anxiety and tension by activating the parasympathetic nervous system.

3. Helps the body prepare for rest, resulting in better sleep quality.

D. Nadi Shodhana (alternate nostril breathing)

Nadi Shodhana, also known as alternating nostril breathing, is an ancient pranayama (yogic breathing) practice for balancing the body's energies and relaxing the mind. Breathing through one nostril at a time helps to balance the brain's right and left hemispheres, reduce stress, and increase mental clarity.

Instructions:

1. Sit in a comfortable position, spine straight and shoulders relaxed.
2. Use your right thumb to seal your right nostril.
3. Inhale deeply from the left nostril.
4. Close your left nostril with your right ring finger, then release your right nose.
5. Exhale gently and thoroughly from your right nostril.
6. Inhale deeply via your right nostril.
7. Close your right nostril while releasing your left.
8. Exhale gently and thoroughly from your left nostril.
9. Repeat for 5–10 minutes, concentrating on the flow of breath.

Benefits:

1. Reduces stress and anxiety by encouraging a sense of balance.
2. Improves lung capacity and respiratory function.
3. Enhances mental clarity, focus, and concentration.

E. Resonant or Coherent Breathing

Resonant breathing is the practice of breathing slowly and rhythmically to synchronize the body's natural rhythms and promote relaxation. This approach is similar to diaphragmatic breathing but focuses on reducing the breath rate to five to six breaths per minute, which has been demonstrated to enhance heart rate variability and reduce stress.

Instructions:

1. Sit comfortably, back straight and shoulders relaxed.
2. Inhale gently through your nose for 5 seconds.
3. Exhale gently through your nose for five seconds.
4. Repeat this pattern for 5-10 minutes, concentrating on calm, continuous breathing.

Benefits:

1. Improves heart rate variability, which indicates a healthy autonomic nervous system.
2. Reduces anxiety and tension by encouraging profound relaxation.
3. Improves general emotional well-being and mental clarity.

F. Breath Counting

Breath counting is a simple but effective practice for relaxing the mind and relieving stress. It entails counting each inhale and exhale, which helps to direct the mind's attention away from unpleasant ideas and onto the present moment.

Instructions:

1. Sit comfortably, with your back straight.
2. Close your eyes and take a deep inhale through your nose.
3. As you exhale, quietly count "one."
4. On your next inhale, count "two" as you breathe in.
5. Continue to count each breath until you reach ten. Once you've reached ten, start over at one.
6. If your mind wanders, softly return your attention to the breathing and counting procedure.

Benefits:

1. Keeps the mind focused on the breath, which helps to relax.
2. Encourages mindfulness and being present in the moment.
3. Reduces stress and anxiety by inducing deep relaxation.

Deep breathing exercises are easy, effective, and adaptable practices that anybody, anywhere, can do to relieve muscle tension and calm the nervous system. From diaphragmatic breathing to alternate nostril breathing, these techniques engage the body's inherent relaxation mechanisms, reducing anxiety and promoting a sense of calm and well-being. By adopting deep breathing into your everyday routine, you may reduce stress, relieve pain, and improve your overall mental and physical health.

2. Progressive Muscular Relaxation (PMR)

Progressive Muscle Relaxation (PMR) is a very efficient technique that involves systematically tensing and relaxing various muscle groups throughout the body. PMR, invented by Dr. Edmund Jacobson in the 1930s, is based on the idea that physical relaxation can have a calming impact on the mind, and vice versa. Individuals can relieve physical strain as well as mental stress and worry by actively tightening (contracting) and then relaxing each muscle group.

The approach has two main components:

❖ Tension involves actively tensing a muscle group for a few seconds.

❖ Relaxation is the process of releasing tension and focusing on a feeling of relaxation for an extended length of time.

This cycle of tension and relaxation can help the body distinguish between tension and relaxation, making it easier to identify and manage stress over time. PMR is very beneficial for people suffering from chronic pain, muscle stiffness, anxiety, and stress-related disorders.

PMR works to stop the cycle of muscle tension and stress. When a person is apprehensive or stressed, the body typically responds by tightening muscles in numerous regions. This involuntary muscular contraction is part of the body's "fight or flight" reaction, which serves to prepare it for action. However, when this tension becomes persistent, it can cause discomfort and even worsen pre-existing pain, such as sciatica, back pain, or tension headaches.

Individuals who practice PMR can reduce the consequences of prolonged muscle tension. The practice trains the body to detect and release unwanted tension, which can help alleviate pain and anxiety. The relaxation that occurs after each muscular contraction also activates the parasympathetic nervous system (the "rest and digest" system), which promotes relaxation and healing.

Benefits of Progressive Muscle Relaxation:

1. Reduces Muscle Tension: One of the primary benefits of PMR is the release of physical muscle tension, which can help with discomfort, particularly in tight areas like the lower back, neck, shoulders, and hips. This is especially useful for people who have sciatica, as tight muscles can increase nerve discomfort.

2. Reduces Anxiety and Stress: By focusing on the process of tensing and releasing muscles, PMR assists individuals in managing the physical symptoms of anxiety and stress. It improves relaxation by shifting focus away from negative thoughts and toward body sensations.

3. Improves Sleep: Studies have shown that regular PMR practice helps people fall asleep faster and sleep deeper and more restfully. The relaxation it delivers can help to relieve physical tightness and mental tension, which can often interfere with getting a good night's sleep.

4. Increases Body Awareness: PMR helps people become more aware of where stress is stored in their bodies. Some people, for example, may unconsciously clench their jaws or hold tension in their shoulders. Increased awareness of these patterns enables people to make proactive efforts to correct them before they cause discomfort or pain.

5. Improves Overall Relaxation: The intentional concentration on tensing and releasing muscle groups generates a deep level of relaxation, making it simpler for the body to recuperate from physical activity or stress. This relaxation extends beyond the muscles to the nervous system, which promotes general mental health.

How to Practice Progressive Muscle Relaxation

PMR can be done in a calm, comfortable setting where you will not be distracted. It does not require any additional equipment, though some people like to lie down on a mat or soft surface for practice. Here's a step-by-step guide for performing PMR.

Step 1: Find a quiet space

Choose a quiet, comfortable area where you can unwind without distractions. This could be a quiet space at home or a serene corner of the office. To completely participate in the technique, you must first feel safe and comfortable.

Step 2: Sit or lie down comfortably

PMR can be performed while sitting or lying down, as long as you are relaxed. If you're lying down, make sure your body is supported by a hard surface and that your head, neck, and spine are in alignment.

Step 3: Take several deep breaths

Take a few deep breaths before starting to tighten your muscles. Inhale deeply through your nose, allowing your lungs to fully expand, then gently exhale through your mouth. This will help to quiet your nervous system and prepare you for the relaxation process.

Step 4: Begin with the lower body

❖ Begin from your feet and gradually work your way up toward your head, concentrating on one muscle group at a time. The steps for each muscle group are as follows:
❖ Inhale and contract the muscles in a certain section of your body. Hold the tension for approximately 5-10 seconds. Tighten the muscles without straining or producing pain.
❖ Exhale and release the tension in your muscles. Concentrate on the sensation of relaxation as your muscles soften and loosen. Try to maintain a relaxed state for at least 15-20 seconds, focusing on the contrast between tension and relaxation.
❖ Move on to the next muscle group: Once one group of muscles has been relaxed, move on to the next. Repeat the method for each part of the body.

Here's a breakdown of the muscle groups to target:

❖ Curl your toes and contract the muscles in your feet. Hold for 5-10 seconds and then release. Notice the contrast between tension and relaxation.

❖ Tighten your calf muscles by pointing your toes and flexing them. Hold for a few seconds and then release.

❖ Firm your thighs by squeezing them together. Hold then release.

❖ Suck in and tighten your abdominal muscles. Hold for a few seconds then release.

❖ Take a big breath in and tighten your chest muscles. Hold, then breathe out and relax.

❖ Close your fists and strain your forearms, then relax and let go.

❖ Shrug your shoulders up to your ears, then hold and release. Then, gently tilt your head from side to side.

❖ Tighten your facial muscles by scrunching your forehead, squinting your eyes, and clenching your jaw. Hold for a few seconds then release.

Step 5: Repeat the process

After completing the whole body scan, you can repeat the process to deepen your relaxation. Some people like to target a specific muscle group that is particularly tight or stiff, such as the neck or lower back.

Step 6: Finish with deep breathing

After you've finished the relaxation cycle, take a few minutes to breathe deeply and relax. Inhale gently through your nose, extending your abdomen, then exhale slowly through your mouth. Allow your body to completely relax and enjoy the sense of serenity you've achieved.

Progressive Muscle Relaxation is a great way to relieve muscle tension and calm the nervous system. Whether you're dealing with chronic pain, or tension, or simply want to relax more, PMR can help you achieve a deeper level of serenity and mental clarity. By adding PMR into your daily routine, you can become more aware of your body's stress and learn to release it deliberately, improving long-term relaxation, pain alleviation, and mental health.

3. Meditation & Mindfulness

Meditation and mindfulness are effective strategies for relaxing the neurological system and lowering muscle tension. These strategies not only aid with stress management but also provide a comprehensive approach to addressing the physical and emotional issues that contribute to chronic pain, such as sciatica.

Meditation and mindfulness help people focus their attention and regulate their emotional responses to stress and discomfort. When we are agitated or in pain, our sympathetic nervous system is triggered, triggering the fight-or-flight reaction. This raises heart rate, shallow breathing, and muscle tension, all of which can exacerbate discomfort and make it difficult to relax.

Meditation and mindfulness, on the other hand, stimulate the parasympathetic nervous system, which regulates the body's rest-and-digest condition. This shift promotes slower breathing, a lower heart rate, and the release of endorphins, which are natural compounds in the body that relieve pain and promote relaxation. These techniques assist lessen the impression of stress and discomfort by fostering awareness of the present moment and encouraging nonjudgmental acceptance, allowing the body to let go of tension and regain equilibrium more easily.

A. Meditation Techniques to Reduce Muscle Tension

Meditation can take many different forms, but they all entail the development of focused attention, awareness, and relaxation. The following are some popular meditation techniques for calming the nervous system, reducing muscle tension, and increasing mental clarity.

1. Guided Meditation

Guided meditation is an ideal choice for beginners since it entails listening to the voice of a teacher or instructor as they lead you through a series of visualizations or relaxation techniques. Guided meditations for muscle tension and sciatica may include body scans, deep relaxation, and imagery that aids healing and pain reduction.

Instructions:

1. Find a quiet, comfortable spot to sit or lie down.
2. To relax, close your eyes and take several deep breaths.
3. Listen to a guided meditation on an app, on YouTube, or in a recorded session. Concentrate on the instructor's voice as they walk you through the process of relaxing each muscle group, beginning with your toes and working your way up to your head.
4. As you go, imagine each part of your body becoming warm and relaxed. This can help relieve tension in the back, legs, and hips, which are commonly impacted by sciatica.

Guided meditation frequently focuses on relieving mental tension and stress, which can present as physical tightness. It is especially useful for people who struggle to relax on their own.

2. Body Scan Meditation

Body scan meditation is a mindfulness practice in which you mentally scan your body to identify areas of tension or discomfort. This technique promotes nonjudgmental awareness and acceptance of your body's sensations, which can help relieve stress and muscle tightness.

Instructions:

1. Lie down in a comfortable posture, either on your back or seated, and close your eyes.
2. Focus your attention on your breath. Consider the sensation of air going in and out of your body.
3. Begin with your toes, noting any feelings of warmth, tightness, or discomfort. Recognize the sensations without judgment, and then intentionally relax the area.
4. Move gradually up the body, scanning each section (feet, legs, hips, abdomen, chest, arms, neck, and head). As you become aware of regions of tension, work on relaxing them.
5. If you have any pain or tightness, try to soften and release it with each breath.

This sort of meditation not only relieves muscle tension but also helps people develop more body awareness, which is necessary for identifying and treating sources of pain and suffering.

3. Loving-kindness Meditation (Metta)

Loving-kindness meditation, also known as Metta, aims to cultivate compassion and positive thoughts for oneself and others. This practice can help minimize the emotional burden of chronic pain and stress by creating a sense of serenity, warmth, and kindness, all of which serve to relax the nervous system.

Instructions:

1. Sit comfortably with your eyes closed, then take a few deep breaths to focus yourself.
2. Begin by quietly repeating expressions of love and compassion, such as:
   - *"May I be happy?"*
   - *"May I be peaceful?"*
   - *"May I be free from suffering?"*
   - *"May I be healthy?"*
3. As you repeat these phrases, envision sending loving energy to yourself, filling your body with warmth and compassion.
4. Once you've spent some time focused on yourself, you can gradually extend your wishes to others, beginning with close ones and progressing to all living beings.

Loving-kindness meditation promotes good feelings, which improves how we deal with discomfort. Individuals can transform their thinking by focusing on compassion and kindness, resulting in a more relaxed mood and lower levels of stress and suffering.

B. *Mindfulness Techniques to help reduce Muscle Tension and Stress*

Mindfulness is the practice of being completely present and engaged in the moment without passing judgment. It entails observing one's thoughts, feelings, and body sensations as they occur rather than reacting to them. In the context of muscle tension and pain treatment, mindfulness helps people become more aware of tiny changes in their bodies, allowing them to relieve tension before it becomes chronic.

1. Mindful Breathing

Mindful breathing is one of the most basic and effective strategies to alleviate stress and muscle tension. Individuals can refocus their attention away from discomfort and into a state of serenity by focusing on their breathing. Breathing gently and deeply also helps the body relax and relieve tension.

Instructions:

1. Sit or lie in a comfortable position.
2. Pay attention to your breathing, experiencing the sensation of the air moving in and out of your body.
3. Inhale through your nose, letting your belly rise, and exhale gently through your mouth.
4. If your thoughts begin to wander, softly return your focus to the breath without judgment.

Mindful breathing can be very helpful when dealing with sciatica or other chronic pain. It helps to shift the attention from agony to relaxation, making it easier to manage pain and lessen muscle tension.

2. Mindful Movement

Mindful movement entails engaging in gentle physical activity while keeping completely aware of the body's sensations and movements. This practice is quite similar to yoga, tai chi, and qigong, all of which emphasize slow, deliberate movements mixed with breath awareness.

Instructions:

1. Walking, stretching, or yoga are examples of slow, gentle activities that you can do comfortably. As you move, focus your complete attention on the sensation of your body in motion.
2. Concentrate on each breath and how it flows with your motions. Pay attention to regions of tension and work on softening them with each inhale and exhale.

This technique not only relieves physical stress but also raises awareness of habitual patterns of tension in the body, allowing for deeper relaxation.

Mindful movement can help people connect more profoundly with their bodies and become more aware of where they retain stress, allowing them to release it gradually over time.

The Advantages of Meditation and Mindfulness for Sciatica Relief

Meditation and mindfulness provide several benefits for people suffering from sciatica and chronic pain:

1. Pain Reduction: By focusing on the present moment and adopting a nonjudgmental attitude toward pain, people can change their perception of it. Meditation and mindfulness help to lessen the intensity of pain by encouraging calm and emotional detachment.

2. Muscle Relaxation: These techniques activate the parasympathetic nerve system, which causes the body to relax, lowering muscle tension and aiding healing.

3. Improved Sleep: Chronic pain can disrupt sleep, but meditation and mindfulness have been demonstrated to improve sleep quality by lowering tension and increasing relaxation.

4. Emotional Regulation: Meditation and mindfulness help people develop emotional resilience, allowing them to manage better the stress and frustration that chronic pain often brings.

Meditation and mindfulness are extremely efficient methods of relaxing the neurological system and relieving physical tension. Individuals suffering from sciatica and other types of chronic pain can improve their general well-being by implementing these activities into their daily lives. Whether through guided meditation, body scans, loving-kindness practices, or mindful breathing and movement, these techniques provide simple, natural ways to improve relaxation, relieve pain, and recover control of one's body and mind.

4. Heat and Cold Therapy

Heat and cold therapy are popular, low-cost, non-invasive therapies for pain relief, muscle relaxation, and improving recovery from various injuries or diseases, including sciatica. Both therapies function by regulating blood flow, decreasing inflammation, and promoting muscular relaxation. Understanding how and when to apply each therapy allows you to successfully reduce discomfort, enhance mobility, and speed up the healing process.

A. Heat Therapy

Heat treatment works by boosting blood flow to the area of discomfort or tension, which relaxes stiff muscles, alleviates pain, and promotes healing. When heat is delivered to a specific area, the blood vessels dilate, increasing circulation and allowing more oxygen and nutrients to enter the tissues. This can also aid in washing out toxins and metabolic waste that may have accumulated in the muscles and tissues, accelerating healing.

How heat therapy works:

1. Heat is good at relaxing stiff muscles, increasing suppleness, and reducing muscle spasms. It is very effective for chronic pain, stiffness, and muscle tightness.
2. Heat causes blood vessels to enlarge, allowing for enhanced circulation. This increased blood flow helps deliver oxygen and nutrients to the muscles, hastening the mending process.
3. Heat can help relieve pain by calming painful muscles, decreasing joint stiffness, and increasing relaxation. It also promotes the release of endorphins, the body's natural pain relievers.
4. Heat can enhance tissue flexibility, making joints and muscles easier to move and stretch. This is useful for disorders like sciatica, in which flexibility and movement may be hindered due to muscular tension.

Types of Heat Therapy:

1. Moist heat, such as warm towels, heat packs, or a warm shower, is particularly good for deeper muscular tissues. Moisture improves heat penetration and keeps the heat source warm for longer.
2. Dry heat sources, such as heating pads, electric blankets, and heated rice bags, are useful and can provide rapid comfort. However, they may not go as deep into the muscles as moist heat.
3. Immersing the body in warm water relaxes muscles and reduces stress. Epsom salts in the bath can boost the relaxing effect by containing magnesium, which relaxes muscles and relieves pain.
4. Heat wraps or patches are often adhesive patches that can be applied directly to the affected part of the skin. They deliver continuous, moderate heat for hours and are particularly effective for alleviating localized pain.

When to use heat therapy:

1. Chronic Muscular Tension: Heat is effective for relieving chronic pain and muscular stiffness. Heat helps to stretch tight muscles and alleviate joint stiffness, which is beneficial for conditions such as sciatica, arthritis, and fibromyalgia.
2. Before Exercise or Stretching: Using heat to warm up muscles helps them become more flexible and less prone to injury.

3. Heat is also useful for general relaxation and stress alleviation, which can help alleviate muscle tension produced by stress or anxiety.

Precautions for heat therapy:

* Heat should not be applied to regions of swelling or inflammation, since it can exacerbate the disease.
* Avoid applying heat to exposed wounds or cuts.
* If you have diabetes or poor circulation, see your doctor before using heat therapy because it can damage the body's capacity to regulate temperature.

B. Cold Therapy

Cold treatment, also known as cryotherapy, is the process of putting ice or cold packs on a specific part of the body to reduce inflammation, numb pain, and limit blood flow. Cold has a numbing effect that can temporarily reduce pain by inhibiting the activation of nerve endings in the affected region. It also reduces swelling by constricting blood arteries, slowing the flow of fluid to the area.

How cold therapy works:

1. Cold therapy helps to decrease inflammation by decreasing blood flow to the affected area. This is especially useful for acute injuries, such as strains, sprains, or flare-ups of disorders like sciatica, where swelling can exacerbate pain.
2. Cold therapy operates as a natural anesthetic, numbing the area and dulling pain signals to the brain. This can provide quick, temporary relief from sharp, excruciating pain.
3. Cold therapy prevents swelling by restricting blood vessels, reducing the flow of fluids to the affected area, and limiting tissue damage in the early stages of injury.
4. Applying ice to the affected area might lessen muscle spasms and stress by slowing down muscular activity, thus breaking the pain cycle.

Types of cold therapy:

1. Ice Packs: A simple and effective way is to wrap an ice pack in a cloth or towel. To avoid frostbite, do not place ice directly on the skin. Ice packs can be used for 15-20 minutes every few hours for the first 48-72 hours following an injury or flare-up.
2. Cold Gel Packs: These are reusable gel packs that can be frozen and used on affected regions. They are flexible and can adjust to the body's contours, making them suitable for treating localized discomfort like sciatica or back pain.

3. Ice massage involves rubbing an ice cube or ice pack in a circular motion over the affected area to provide immediate relief from pain and inflammation. This method is successful in smaller, more localized areas.

4. Cold Compression Wraps: These wraps combine cold therapy and mild compression to reduce swelling and provide continuous relief. They are most typically used for joint injuries, but they can also be used to treat muscle pain.

When to use cold therapy:

1. Cold therapy is most effective right after an injury or flare-up of inflammation. For example, if you have sudden sciatica pain or a muscle strain, applying cold can assist reduce swelling and relieve discomfort.

2. Cold therapy is beneficial for reducing muscle spasms, especially when applied shortly after the muscle begins to cramp. It helps to lessen the muscle's involuntary contraction.

3. If you overexert yourself during an exercise or workout, cold therapy can help reduce inflammation and muscle discomfort.

Precautions for cold therapy

- ❖ To avoid frostbite or tissue damage, do not apply cold for more than 20 minutes at a time.
- ❖ If you have poor circulation, do not use cold therapy because it may worsen your condition.
- ❖ Never apply ice to exposed skin; instead, use a barrier such as a towel or cloth to avoid direct contact with the ice.

Alternating heat and cold therapy (contrast therapy)

In other circumstances, alternating between heat and cold therapy can produce even more beneficial results. This procedure, known as contrast therapy, consists of providing heat for a specified period, followed by cold therapy, and repeating the cycle. The alternating impacts of heat and cold increase blood flow, reduce inflammation and promote healing in a balanced manner.

How it works:

1. Heat First: Apply heat to the affected area for 10-15 minutes to increase blood flow and relax muscles.
2. Cold Therapy: Following the heat, apply 10-15 minutes of cold therapy to reduce inflammation and numb discomfort.
3. Repeat: Alternate between heat and cold for 30-45 minutes, finishing with cold therapy to reduce swelling.

Heat and cold therapy are effective methods for treating muscle tension, discomfort, and inflammation, particularly in disorders such as sciatica. Heat relaxes muscles and improves circulation, whilst cold reduces swelling and numbs acute discomfort. Individuals who use both methods correctly can get improved pain relief, faster healing, and increased mobility. Always evaluate the nature of your ailment and listen to your body when determining which therapy to use, and if required, consult a healthcare expert for more personalized recommendations.

5. Aromatherapy and Essential Oil

Aromatherapy is an ancient therapeutic practice that uses natural plant extracts known as essential oils to improve physical, emotional, and psychological well-being. Aromatherapy, which harnesses the power of scent, can influence both the mind and the body, helping to reduce stress, relieve muscle tension, and relax the neurological system. Aromatherapy essential oils are derived from a variety of plant parts, including flowers, leaves, roots, bark, and seeds, and each oil has distinct advantages.

Aromatherapy works in a variety of ways to promote muscular relaxation and overall well-being. The aroma of essential oils is breathed through the nose and processed by the olfactory system before being transmitted to the brain, including the limbic system, which is in charge of emotions, memories, and certain body processes such as heart rate and blood pressure. This is why fragrances may have such a strong impact on our emotions and physical state. When used correctly, aromatherapy can assist in relieving stress, and muscle tension, and induce a state of relaxation that promotes healing.

Aromatherapy works by employing the sense of smell to elicit physiological reactions that aid in relaxation and healing. When you inhale the aroma of an essential oil, the molecules travel to the brain's olfactory bulb, where they connect with the limbic system. The limbic system, also known as the "emotional brain," regulates mood, stress, and heart rate.

Essential oils can stimulate the limbic system by:

1. Reducing tension and anxiety: Many essential oils have relaxing effects that help you relax.
2. Alleviating pain: Some essential oils, such as eucalyptus or peppermint, have analgesic (pain-relieving) characteristics that can aid with muscle soreness.
3. Boosting circulation: Certain oils, such as rosemary, can help boost blood flow, which aids in muscle recuperation.
4. Regulating the nervous system: Oils such as lavender and chamomile can assist in balancing the nervous system and promote tranquility.

The oils can be utilized in a variety of ways, including inhalation, topical application (diluted with a carrier oil), and a warm bath. Below, we'll look at some of the most popular essential oils for soothing the nervous system and alleviating muscle tension.

1. Lavender Essential Oil

Lavender is one of the most well-known essential oils because of its powerful relaxing and soothing properties. It is often used in aromatherapy to promote relaxation, sleep, and stress reduction.

Benefits:

1. Lavender is known for its relaxing characteristics, making it an ideal choice for calming the mind and muscles.
2. It can aid with anxiety, stress, and depression by producing calm and emotional stability.
3. It relieves muscle stress by relaxing the body and reducing tension in the neck, shoulders, and back.
4. Lavender contains anti-inflammatory qualities that can help calm aching muscles and alleviate discomfort.

How to use:

1. Inhalation: Place a few drops of lavender oil in a diffuser and inhale deeply. The smell will assist in relaxing your nervous system and lessen anxiety.

2. Topical application: Dilute lavender oil with a carrier oil (such as coconut or almond oil) and gently massage it into tight muscles or tension points.
3. Bath: Pour 5-10 drops of lavender essential oil into a warm bath to help calm your body and mind.

2. Peppermint Essential Oil

Peppermint is known for its energizing and cooling properties, making it great for relieving muscle tension and increasing circulation. This essential oil is a popular choice for treating headaches and muscle stress.

Benefits:

1. Peppermint has a cooling effect that can provide instant relief for stiff, aching muscles.
2. It contains menthol, which has analgesic (pain-relieving) properties, making it ideal for tension headaches, neck discomfort, and back pain.
3. It improves circulation by increasing blood flow to areas of tension, which promotes faster muscle recovery.
4. Peppermint's invigorating scent can also help relieve weariness and increase attentiveness.

How to use:

1. Topical Application: Dilute peppermint oil with carrier oil and apply it directly to tight muscles or the temples to relieve tension headaches. The chilly sensation will assist relax the muscles.
2. Inhalation: Place a few drops in a diffuser to produce a stimulating and energetic environment, perfect for relieving tension and enhancing attention.
3. Cold Compress: Combine a few drops of peppermint oil and water and apply to a cold compress. Apply the compress to your painful muscles for comfort.

3. Eucalyptus Essential Oil

Another effective muscle relief oil is eucalyptus essential oil, which has anti-inflammatory and analgesic qualities. It is notably good for respiratory difficulties, but it can also help with muscle stiffness and blood circulation.

Benefits:

1. Eucalyptus contains strong anti-inflammatory effects that can help relieve swelling and irritation in aching muscles and joints.
2. It provides a cooling effect that can alleviate the discomfort of muscle tightness.

3. The oil is antispasmodic, which means it helps to relieve muscle spasms and tightness, notably in the back, neck, and legs.
4. Eucalyptus essential oil helps promote circulation by increasing blood flow to stiff or painful areas and speeding up muscle recovery.

How to use:

1. Topical application: Mix eucalyptus oil with a carrier oil and massage it into tight muscles, especially in the lower back, neck, and shoulders.
2. Inhalation: Place eucalyptus oil in a diffuser to clear the airways and induce relaxation while also reducing muscle tension.
3. Bath: Add a few drops of eucalyptus oil to a warm bath to help relax the body and relieve muscle stiffness.

4. Chamomile Essential Oil

Chamomile, especially Roman Chamomile, is widely used in aromatherapy due to its relaxing, anti-inflammatory, and calming effects. This oil is ideal for decreasing stress, relaxing the mind, and relieving muscle tightness.

Benefits:

1. Chamomile is known for its relaxing effects on both the mind and body, making it an excellent stress reliever.
2. It contains anti-inflammatory characteristics that can help relieve muscle stiffness and stress, particularly in the neck, shoulders, and lower back.
3. Chamomile is also beneficial in supporting better sleep, which is necessary for muscle healing and overall health.

How to use:

1. Inhalation: Place a few drops of chamomile essential oil in a diffuser to relax the mind and produce a peaceful atmosphere.
2. Topical Application: Massage diluted chamomile oil into aching muscles or use it to ease neck and shoulder stress.
3. Bath: Adding chamomile oil to a warm bath reduces muscle tension and promotes relaxation.

5. Rosemary Essential Oil

Rosemary oil is commonly used to increase circulation, stimulate the nervous system, and relieve pain. Its exhilarating and refreshing scent lifts the mood while relieving muscle tension.

Benefits:

1. Rosemary oil promotes circulation, which helps alleviate muscle tension by increasing blood flow to the affected areas.
2. It contains analgesic qualities, making it useful for relieving pain and suffering, particularly muscle tightness or joint pain.
3. Rosemary also acts as a muscle relaxant, helping to soften tight, stiff muscles.

How to use:

1. Topical Application: Combine rosemary oil and a carrier oil, then massage it into tight muscles or painful regions. It is especially effective for lower back discomfort.
2. Inhalation: Place rosemary oil in a diffuser for a refreshing and invigorating ambiance that also aids with pain treatment.
3. Bath: Add a few drops of rosemary oil to a warm bath to reduce tension and increase circulation.

Aromatherapy and the use of essential oils provide a natural and efficient technique to relax the nervous system and ease muscle tension. Individuals can dramatically improve their entire sense of well-being by using the correct essential oils, such as lavender for relaxation, peppermint for pain treatment, eucalyptus for inflammation, chamomile for stress, or rosemary for circulation. These oils can be used to treat chronic pain, muscle tightness, and stress in a variety of ways, including inhalation, topical application, and baths. Incorporating essential oils into your daily self-care practice will help you relax, recuperate your muscles, and create a tranquil, pain-free atmosphere for healing.

6. Massage and Self-Massage

A massage is a tried-and-true approach for lowering muscle tension, relaxing, and soothing the nervous system. Massage, whether conducted by a professional massage therapist or at home using self-massage techniques, has numerous physical and mental advantages.

Massage works by targeting the body's soft tissues, which include muscles, tendons, and ligaments. Massage improves blood circulation, relieves muscle tension, and stimulates the release of endorphins, the body's natural pain-relieving chemicals. Applying pressure to specific places or areas of tension helps to release muscular knots (trigger points), reduce inflammation, and restore correct muscle length, flexibility, and range of motion.

Massage not only offers physical benefits, but it also has a significant impact on the nervous system. Massage stimulates the parasympathetic nervous system (the "rest and digest" system), which balances the effects of the sympathetic nervous system (the "fight or flight" reaction). This reduces stress, anxiety, and the feeling of pain, promoting relaxation and well-being.

Massage treatments vary in approach and advantages. Some of the most frequent types of therapeutic massage are:

A. Swedish Massage

Swedish massage is one of the most popular types of massage therapy, recognized for its soft, relaxing strokes. It entails extended gliding strokes, kneading, circular motions, and tapping. Swedish massage is effective for promoting overall relaxation, increasing circulation, and relieving superficial muscle tension.

Swedish massage can help relax the muscles in the back and hips that are commonly impacted by sciatica. It is especially efficient at relieving tension in the gluteal and lower back muscles, which can contribute to sciatica symptoms.

B. Deep Tissue Massage

Deep tissue massage applies more forceful pressure to deeper levels of muscle and connective tissue. It targets deeper muscle fibers and tissue to alleviate chronic muscle tension, adhesions, and muscle knots.

Deep tissue massage can help those with sciatica or chronic lower back pain by releasing stiffness in the deep muscles and fascia surrounding the sciatic nerve. Addressing muscle imbalances and limits may help relieve pressure on the sciatic nerve and increase mobility.

C. Myofascial Release:

Myofascial release is a technique for treating the fascia, the connective tissue that surrounds muscles, bones, and organs. This massage technique employs prolonged pressure and mild stretching to alleviate fascial tightness and limitations that can cause muscle discomfort and stiffness.

Tight fascia around the lower back, hips, and thighs can exacerbate the condition. Myofascial release focuses on these areas to decrease tension and increase muscular flexibility, which can lessen pressure on the sciatic nerve.

D. Trigger-Point Therapy:

Trigger point therapy focuses on locating and relaxing tight, hyper-irritable regions of a muscle. These sites frequently refer pain to other parts of the body, resulting in a cycle of tension and discomfort.

People with sciatica frequently have trigger points in their lower backs, hips, and legs. Trigger point therapy works by providing direct pressure to these spots, which helps to release muscle knots and reduces referred pain down the sciatic nerve.

E. Hot Stone Massage

Hot stone massage uses smooth, hot stones that are put on the body or used by the therapist as massage implements. The heat from the stones relaxes muscles and improves circulation, while the stones' weight applies deeper pressure.

The heat from the stones relaxes tight muscles, while the weight of the stones can apply deeper pressure to address deep muscular tension, particularly in the lower back and hips, which are frequently impacted by sciatica.

Benefits of Massage

Professional massage therapy is extremely beneficial, yet it may not be accessible or inexpensive to everyone. Fortunately, self-massage is a simple and affordable technique to reduce muscle tension, relieve pain, and promote relaxation in the comfort of your own home. Self-massage has several significant benefits, including:

1. Convenience and Accessibility: Self-massage can be performed at any time, including during a work break, after a long day, or while watching television. It does not require

an appointment or travel, making it a simple way to relieve muscle tension.

2. Increased Body Awareness: Self-massage helps people become more aware of their bodies and identify areas of tension or discomfort. This improved bodily awareness can assist reduce muscle strain and allow people to adapt their posture and movement patterns to avoid future injuries.

3. Cost-Effectiveness: Regular professional massage treatments can be expensive, but self-massage can deliver equivalent advantages at a lower cost. All you need are simple instruments like massage balls, foam rollers, or even your own hands.

4. Empowerment and Control: Self-massage allows people to take charge of their health and wellness. It lets patients actively manage their pain and suffering by focusing on specific muscle groups or trigger points.

Self-Massage Techniques

Here are several excellent self-massage techniques for lowering muscle tension and relieving pain, particularly in areas frequently affected by sciatica:

❖ **Foam Rolling:** Foam rolling is an effective self-massage technique for major muscular areas including the calves, thighs, and lower back. Rolling slowly over the foam roller will help you release stiffness and enhance flexibility. For sciatica, foam rolling the lower back, hamstrings, and glutes can help relieve tension that may be causing the discomfort. Concentrate on the regions where tightness and discomfort are most noticeable. Roll slowly and pause on sore regions for 20-30 seconds to relieve muscle tension.

❖ **Tennis Ball Massage:** A tennis ball can be used to do more targeted self-massage. Place the ball between your body and a wall or the floor, then gently roll it over areas of tension including your lower back, glutes, and upper thighs. For sciatica, when the piriformis muscle in the gluteal region tightens, it can cause significant sciatica pain. Apply light pressure to the piriformis area with a tennis ball to assist release of tension and relieve strain on your sciatic nerve.

❖ **Handheld Massagers:** Handheld massagers, such as percussion massagers or vibration devices, can help relieve stress in specific regions. Individuals can change the pressure and speed to their desired level of comfort. To relieve sciatica, use a handheld massager on the lower back, hips, and thighs to relax muscle tension. The deep vibrations can reach deeper into the muscles, reducing spasms and improving blood flow.

❖ **Manual Trigger Point Release:** Manually releasing trigger points involves applying direct pressure to specific muscle knots with your fingers, thumbs, or elbows. Apply pressure to the knot for 20-30 seconds, then release. For sciatica, concentrate on the glutes, lower back, and thighs. These locations frequently include trigger points that can lead to sciatica. Apply consistent pressure to the knots with your thumb or fingers, and then slowly release.

Combining Massage and Other Techniques

Self-massage can be used with other treatments like stretching, heat therapy, and breathing exercises to provide the most relief possible. For example, after massaging a stiff muscle, a mild stretch can help to lengthen the fibers and induce relaxation. Furthermore, combining deep breathing with massage can activate the parasympathetic nervous system, which improves the relaxation response.

Massage and self-massage are effective ways to reduce muscle tension, relieve pain, and relax the nervous system. Individuals can take control of their health and get relief from illnesses such as sciatica by learning about the many types of massage and adopting self-massage techniques into their daily practice. Regular massage, whether performed by a professional or at home, helps to preserve muscle flexibility, relieve chronic pain, and improve general well-being.

By implementing these practices into their daily lives, people can successfully soothe their nervous systems and minimize muscle tension. Whether it's deep breathing, meditation, gentle stretching, or heat therapy, each method promotes relaxation, reduces discomfort, and restores a sense of well-being. Consistently applying these strategies can help people relieve chronic pain, reduce stress, and recover control of their bodies and minds.

CHAPTER 6: DEVELOPING A PERSONALIZED SCIATICA RELIEF ROUTINE

How To Include Exercise Into A Daily Or Weekly Schedule

Developing a daily or weekly exercise plan is critical for controlling sciatica and boosting general mobility and strength, particularly for individuals experiencing chronic pain. However, in order to minimize harm, ensure consistency, and achieve long-term outcomes, this process must be approached systematically.

1. Understanding your goals and needs

The first step in creating an effective fitness plan is to identify your goals. Sciatica sufferers frequently seek pain relief and better mobility. This involves minimizing nerve compression, strengthening the muscles around the spine and pelvis, increasing flexibility, and improving balance.

Some people's goals may be more specific, such as building core strength to support the back or developing flexibility to ease tight muscles. For others, it may be about retaining overall independence and avoiding falls. Understanding your specific goals is critical because it allows you to prioritize the activities that will produce the best outcomes.

2. Determine your fitness level

Before developing a routine, you should examine your present fitness level. Sciatica affects people differently; some have severe pain, while others only feel slight discomfort. Your regimen should be structured to meet you where you are and change as you grow.

If you're a beginner, begin with mild, low-impact activities that build flexibility, strength, and balance without aggravating your pain. As your strength and mobility improve, you can gradually ramp up the intensity of the exercises.

For elders or beginners, exercises such as pelvic tilts, standing calf raises, and moderate hamstring stretches can serve as the cornerstone of your practice. If you are at an intermediate or advanced level, planks, wall squats, and side planks can be used to increase strength and stability.

3. Balancing several types of exercises

An effective sciatica routine should include a variety of exercises that address flexibility, strength, balance, and relaxation. Here's how to include these types of exercises in your routine:

❖ *Flexibility exercises:* Flexibility exercises are vital for releasing muscular tension, increasing mobility, and decreasing pressure on the sciatic nerve. Stretches that target the lower back, hips, hamstrings, and piriformis muscles are very beneficial for sciatica. These stretches should be performed at the beginning and conclusion of your workout, or as part of a light warm-up or cool-down.

❖ *Strengthening exercises:* Strengthening the core, back, and leg muscles is critical for supporting the spine and relieving sciatic discomfort. Strong muscles improve posture, alleviate strain on the sciatic nerve, and provide greater overall body support. Strengthening exercises should be done 2-3 times per week to help build and maintain muscular tone without overworking the body.

❖ *Balance exercises:* Balance exercises are important, especially for seniors, because they help reduce falls and enhance overall stability. Because sciatica frequently causes diminished mobility and coordination, focusing on balance exercises might help you restore independence and confidence. Balance exercises should be done 2-3 times per week, increasing gradually as balance improves.

❖ ***Relaxation and breathing techniques:*** Relaxation and breathing techniques are sometimes disregarded, yet they are equally important as physical activities. These techniques help to manage pain, reduce muscle tension, and increase general well-being. These strategies can be used on a regular basis or after each training session to help with rehabilitation and lessen sciatica discomfort.

4. Structure your weekly routine

Now that you understand the many types of workouts and their functions, the next step is to organize them into a feasible weekly regimen. You can accomplish this by developing a specific approach based on your strengths and capabilities; likewise, try arranging them into sessions. On active days, focus on one or two types of exercises per session, giving your body time to recover in between. If discomfort or weariness develops, limit the intensity or frequency of your workouts. Listen to your body and progress at your speed.

Including exercises in your daily or weekly regimen for sciatica relief is an effective approach to managing pain, increasing mobility, and restoring independence. By incorporating flexibility, strength, balance, and relaxation exercises, you may develop a well-rounded, long-term health program. To reap long-term advantages, start slowly, listen to your body, and gradually increase intensity. With consistency, you can successfully relieve sciatica pain and live a more active and independent life.

Tips For Establishing Realistic Objectives And Monitoring Progress

Setting reasonable objectives and tracking progress are critical components of any fitness program, especially while addressing diseases such as sciatica. For those coping with chronic pain, it is critical to set goals that are not only attainable but also motivating and powerful. Proper goal planning keeps you motivated while tracking progress allows you to check your progress and stay committed.

Here are some guidelines for setting realistic objectives and tracking success on your sciatica healing journey:

1. Understand the importance of realistic goals

Before you start making objectives, you should understand why they need to be realistic. For people suffering from sciatica, the goal isn't only to get through the pain or set unrealistic goals. Setting unrealistic expectations can cause irritation, despair, and even damage. The goal should be to progressively increase flexibility, strength, and mobility while minimizing symptoms.

Realistic goals are attainable in the near term and correspond to your overall long-term goals. They look at your current abilities, restrictions, and recovery time. The idea is to enjoy modest victories along the way rather than expecting immediate, spectacular results.

2. Break down larger goals into smaller, manageable steps

When dealing with sciatica, it's natural to feel overwhelmed by the prospect of major recovery. However, it is critical to break down enormous goals into smaller, more manageable ones.

Instead of setting an overarching goal like "Be pain-free in one month," a more practical approach would be to set weekly targets like:

"Complete stretching exercises for 15 minutes each day."
"Increase the number of repetitions of my pelvic tilt exercise."
"Reduce pain level by 2 points on a scale of 1-10 after three weeks of consistent stretching."

Smaller goals help you keep motivated and focused by providing continuous reminders of your work, even if the greater goal appears distant.

3. Use the SMART Goals Framework

The SMART framework is one of the most effective ways to set realistic goals. SMART stands for the following:

Specific: Make your goal clear and concise. Instead of saying "I want to feel better," go with "I want to increase flexibility in my lower back and hips."
Measurable: Make sure your goal can be tracked. Like the following: "I will reduce the time it takes to perform my morning stretches by 5 minutes within a week."
Achievable: Set a goal that you can reach. If walking makes you uncomfortable, don't aim to run a marathon. Begin with achievable goals, such as "Walk for 10 minutes every other day."
Relevant: The goal should be consistent with your overall desire for greater health or pain reduction. For example, "increase core strength to support my lower back and reduce sciatica pain" is directly related to sciatica relief.
Time-bound: Establish a clear timeline. Rather than stating "I want to improve my posture," say "I want to improve my posture by practicing specific exercises for 10 minutes each day for the next 4 weeks."

The SMART framework can help you achieve goals that are clear, actionable, and attainable.

4. Focus on process-oriented goals

It's tempting to become fixated on the outcome, such as "I want to be completely pain-free in a month," but this can lead to frustration. Instead, focus on process-oriented goals, which are centered on the behaviors or habits that will eventually lead to growth.

Examples of process-oriented goals are:
"I will stretch my hamstrings and lower back every morning for 10 minutes."
"I will perform 3 rounds of core strengthening exercises before bed."
"I will focus on deep breathing during each exercise session to reduce tension."

By focusing on the process rather than the end, you are more likely to form good habits that aid in long-term rehabilitation and pain management.

5. Track progress regularly

Setting objectives and tracking progress are both as crucial. It's easy to lose motivation if you don't feel like you're making any progress, but tracking your progress shows that even minor changes are noticeable. Tracking can help you stay motivated, spot trends, and discover which activities are most effective.

Here is how to effectively track your progress:

A. Keep a journal:

Writing down your daily activities, discomfort levels, and how you felt before and after each session might provide useful insights. Record:
Which exercises did you complete?
How many repetitions or sets you did do?
Any obvious changes in pain or flexibility

This logbook can help you spot trends in your recovery process and make changes if something isn't working.

B. Use a pain tracker:

Tracking your pain levels over time can provide you with a clear picture of your progress. Daily, rate your pain from 1 to 10 before and after activity. This allows you to see if the workouts are effective and whether your pain levels are gradually reducing.

C. Take photographs or measurements:

For some people, visual progress can be a powerful incentive. Take photos of yourself regularly and measure key areas such as hamstring flexibility, lower back range of motion, and posture changes. A comparison of before and after images or measurements can be extremely helpful in building confidence.

D. Celebrate small wins:

Celebrate when you attain a tiny milestone! Whether it's raising the number of repetitions or stretching for an extra 5 minutes, recognizing your progress boosts motivation and maintains the habit of consistency.

6. Adjust goals based on progress

As you track your success, be willing to change your goals. Some goals may seem overly ambitious, while others may appear to be too simple. Don't be hesitant to reassess and adjust your goals based on how you feel.

For example, if your objective was to stretch for 10 minutes each day but you've observed an increase in flexibility, you can extend your stretching time to 15 minutes or incorporate additional stretches into your routine. If you're having trouble completing your exercises, it's fine to back off and alter your goals to match your present ability.

7. Seek professional guidance

Working with a physical therapist or trainer who specializes in injury rehabilitation can help you set realistic goals for your sciatica treatment. A specialist can evaluate your present abilities, offer appropriate workouts, and assist you avoid frequent mistakes that could aggravate your disease.

They can also help you create a more personalized and effective goal-setting technique.

8. Be patient and kind to yourself

Recovery from sciatica is frequently a slow process, with setbacks typical. It's critical to be patient with yourself and understand that progress may take time. Don't be disheartened if you don't achieve your goals right away—this is part of the healing process. The key is to maintain consistency and alter your expectations based on your recovery progress.

Setting realistic objectives and tracking progress are critical elements in treating sciatica. You can retain a sense of success and motivation by breaking down major goals into smaller, manageable tasks, focusing on the process, and recognizing even minor victories. Regularly documenting your pain levels, stretching regimens, and milestones ensures you're on the right course to recovery. Most importantly, be patient and adaptable in your approach; over time, you'll notice that persistent effort and wise goal setting may make a big difference in controlling sciatica pain and improving quality of life.

Changing Routines Based On Pain Levels And Improvements

When dealing with sciatica pain, it is critical to personalize workout programs to each individual's pain level and progression. Sciatica is a disorder that can cause a wide range of symptoms, from minor pains to severe pain. Learning how to alter routines based on pain levels and progress is critical for properly managing sciatica through exercise. This method not only promotes safe healing but also ensures that activities continue to be effective while not increasing symptoms.

Before delving into how to modify activities, it's critical to understand how pain levels change and how they should affect exercise choices.

1. Mild pain is often described as a dull ache or little discomfort. It is acceptable while moving and may not interfere with normal activities. People in minor discomfort may usually undertake most activities without difficulty, however they should be cautious of their motions to prevent exacerbating the disease.

2. Moderate discomfort may feel sharper or more constant, making some motions painful. It may cause tightness in the lower back, legs, or hips, which can impede mobility. Exercise can still be good at this stage, but it requires more

caution and may result in slower improvement. Modifying activities to accommodate pain levels is critical.

3. Severe sciatica pain is strong and often incapacitating, making even the most basic activities difficult. Bending, twisting, and sitting may exacerbate symptoms at this time. Focus on mild movements, stretches, and strengthening exercises to relieve sciatic nerve strain. High-intensity or strenuous exercises should be avoided during this time.

How to Customize Exercises based on Pain Level

Adapting exercises to pain levels entails determining when to adapt, lower intensity, or discontinue. Here are some guidelines to help you with this process:

For mild pain:

Individuals who are in modest pain may usually execute the majority of workouts. However, it is critical to monitor how the body responds, as some activities may produce temporary discomfort.

❖ If the pain is manageable, now is the time to work on strength and flexibility. Exercises such as pelvic tilts, half crunches, and moderate stretches are good at this point. Aim to progressively increase the number of repetitions or the length.

❖ Exercises that strengthen the core, lower back, and legs will assist support the spine and relieve strain on the sciatic nerve. It's critical to avoid overexertion; if pain persists after an activity, lessen the intensity for the following session.

❖ While exercises like wall squats and bridges are great for strengthening, make sure your movements are moderate and controlled. Sudden, abrupt movements might worsen sciatica pain.

For moderate pain:

At this point, it's critical to be extra cautious with exercises, focusing on strategies that don't strain the body. The goal should be to reduce pressure on the sciatic nerve while also increasing circulation, flexibility, and muscle engagement.

❖ Instead of performing full repetitions, shorten the range of action or execute fewer repetitions. Standing calf raises, for example, can be performed with a limited range of motion or only partial raises to avoid overstretching or worsening soreness.

❖ Sciatica is frequently associated with hip and lower back tightness. Stretches such as knee-to-opposite shoulder, piriformis, and hamstring stretches can assist the release of tight muscles without overworking them. To avoid muscle strain, practice these stretches carefully and hold them for 15-30 seconds each.

❖ Chairs or walls can provide support during workouts such as standing on one leg or executing hip abduction. This decreases the danger of balance problems while still giving the benefits of muscle training.

For severe pain:

Severe sciatica pain necessitates extreme caution. Exercises should be low-intensity, with an emphasis on regaining mobility and lowering inflammation rather than increasing strength. The goal at this stage is to alleviate discomfort and increase mobility with mild, low-impact motions.

❖ Exercises like cat-cow positions, child's pose, and lower back rotations are excellent for relieving tension without stressing the body. They should be carried out with caution and avoided if any movement produces severe pain.

❖ Deep breathing techniques (such as diaphragmatic breathing) can assist relieve pain and induce calm. Breathing exercises assist minimize stress, which can worsen muscle tension, thereby alleviating sciatica pain.

❖ At this stage, shorter, more frequent sessions are preferable to longer, more intensive workouts. To progressively improve flexibility and lessen tension, perform 5-10 minutes of easy stretching or relaxation exercises many times per day.

❖ Exercises including lying down or relaxing in supported positions might help relieve lower back tension. When performed correctly, exercises such as lying hamstring stretches or hip openers might be effective.

How to adapt exercises as improvements occur

As the pain improves over time, people can gradually increase the intensity and complexity of their exercises. This advancement should continue to prioritize safety and be gradual to minimize injury.

1. Gradual increase in intensity: As discomfort subsides, gradually include previously avoided exercises. Begin by performing them with a limited range of motion or fewer repetitions, gradually increasing as comfort and strength increase. For example, when the individual gains confidence, they may advance from partial crunches to complete crunches, or from modified planks to standard planks.

2. Incorporate strengthening exercises: Core and lower body strengthening exercises should be added to the plan as flexibility and mobility improve. Bridges, side planks, and

wall squats are good exercises for strengthening the muscles that support the spine. Strengthening exercises like the gluteal stretch and straight leg raises can help minimize sciatic nerve irritation while also improving posture and stability.

3. Use progress tracking: Monitor discomfort, mobility, and strength improvements on a regular basis. Routines should be adjusted as circumstances change. If there is a clear improvement, the exercises can be increased in intensity or length. Documenting progress also helps to motivate people by reminding them of how far they've come and the benefits of hard work.

4. Periodically reevaluate and adapt: It is critical to reassess the pain level on a regular basis and modify the regimen as needed. Just because there have been improvements does not rule out the possibility of fresh pain. A program that is too severe at any given point may cause a flare-up, so be adaptable and change accordingly.

Adapting sciatica cure exercises based on pain levels and progress is a dynamic process that necessitates a thorough understanding of the body's reaction to movement. Individuals can develop an exercise regimen that not only relieves sciatica but also promotes long-term health and independence by assessing pain, modifying intensity, and progressively increasing difficulty as progress is made. With constant effort and proper adaption, persons suffering from sciatica can restore mobility and lessen their dependency on pain medication, ultimately improving their quality of life.

CONCLUSION

Sciatica can be a very painful and restrictive ailment, but it does not have to control your life. With the appropriate workouts and routines, you can not only cure sciatica pain but also improve mobility, flexibility, and strength. The techniques detailed in this book provide a realistic and accessible approach to managing sciatica, particularly for beginners and seniors, so you can begin your journey to relief and recovery immediately.

You should now be able to identify the causes and symptoms of sciatica. The key to overcoming sciatica, whether caused by a herniated disc, spinal stenosis, or tight muscles, is to recognize the value of focused exercises that strengthen and stretch the muscles that support your lower back, hips, and legs. Incorporating these exercises into your everyday regimen can not only relieve pain but also keep it from reoccurring.

One of the most essential ideas in this book is that exercise is more than just pain treatment; it also improves general well-being. Maintaining a schedule of modest, safe workouts, especially for seniors, can considerably enhance mobility and independence and lower the chance of falling. The ability to conduct daily duties with less pain, or even no pain at all, restores a sense of control and independence.

When dealing with sciatica, it is critical to understand that relief will not occur overnight. Patience and persistence are essential, and recognizing that rehabilitation is a lengthy process will help you achieve long-term success. The exercises in this book were carefully selected to provide a gentle beginning to sciatica therapy. They concentrate on strengthening the core, increasing flexibility, and extending the muscles surrounding the spine, hips, and legs. This guarantees that the exercises target the major areas responsible for sciatica pain while being accessible to those just beginning their path to relief.

Gentle warm-up activities are very useful in preparing the body for more specific motions. Warming up helps to activate muscles, improve circulation, and lower the risk of injury. Taking the time to warm up before commencing your workout and cooling down afterward is critical for treating sciatica.

As you implement these exercises into your regimen, you will see changes not only in your mobility but also in your general strength and flexibility. A strong core is essential for supporting the spine and relieving strain on the sciatic nerve. The core exercises recommended in this book, such as pelvic tilts, half crunches, and planks, will help you build the muscle power required to support your lower back.

Exercises such as hip abduction, clamshell, and hamstring stretches relieve muscle stiffness that might lead to sciatica. Muscle stiffness, especially in the glutes, hamstrings, and lower back, can compress the sciatic nerve and exacerbate discomfort. Stretching these areas regularly will assist improve mobility and relieve nerve pressure, hence alleviating pain and discomfort.

By addressing the underlying causes of sciatica with these specific exercises, you can not only ease pain but also avoid future flare-ups. Strengthening the muscles that support the spine and hips offers a solid foundation for stability and lowers the probability of nerve compression. Stretching also increases the flexibility required to maintain appropriate posture, which reduces stress on the sciatic nerve.

One of the most empowering things you can do for yourself is develop a specific sciatica relief program. In Chapter 6, we spoke about how to customize your exercise routine to meet your specific needs, pain levels, and goals. The exercises in this book are versatile enough to be adapted for beginners, seniors, or people of varied fitness levels. Whether you're starting from a place of severe pain or merely want to manage occasional flare-ups, the idea is to start softly and gradually increase the intensity as your body adjusts to the movements.

Tracking your development is also significant because it allows you to observe how you're improving over time. It might be as easy as noticing how much less discomfort you feel after working out or how much more mobility you have. These modest triumphs will act as encouragement to stick to your routine, especially when the discomfort feels overwhelming.

Consistency in your exercises, combined with patience and perseverance, will produce the long-term benefits you seek.

Pain is crucial to remember that sciatica can be a reoccurring condition, particularly if pain is caused by a structural issue such as a herniated disc. In such circumstances, it is critical to remain proactive in treating the illness. Regular exercise, combined with proper posture, body mechanics, and maybe other complementary therapies such as massage or physical therapy, can all help you stay symptom-free.

It is vital to be aware of how your body responds to specific movements. If you experience a major increase in pain or discomfort, you should reconsider your regimen and seek medical attention. Sciatica relief is a comprehensive procedure that includes both activity and paying close attention to how your body is functioning.

While exercise is an important aspect of controlling sciatica, you should also evaluate how other lifestyle variables influence your pain and recovery. Maintaining a healthy weight, avoiding prolonged sitting, and maintaining proper posture can all help to prevent strain on the lower back and sciatic nerve. Simple modifications, such as standing up more often, using ergonomic furniture, or modifying your sleeping posture, can have a significant impact on your overall health.

It's also crucial to be aware of how stress and tension might aggravate sciatica. Incorporating relaxation techniques into your daily routine, such as deep breathing exercises or meditation, can not only help you manage discomfort but will also improve mental health and recovery.

To summarize, sciatica relief is a process that demands patience, consistency, and the appropriate technique. The exercises and strategies described in this book provide a comprehensive and reasonable solution for relieving chronic sciatica pain and increasing mobility. Whether you are a beginner, a senior, or suffering from long-term sciatica, there is hope for healing.

By taking charge of your sciatica with these moderate exercises and a specific routine, you're making a significant investment in your health and well-being. Remember that the route to a pain-free life is within grasp, and with patience and perseverance, you may reclaim the freedom and quality of life that sciatica may have taken away.